WARD LOCK

FAMILY HEALTH GUIDE

CW00401851

ARTHRITIS
& RHEUMATISM

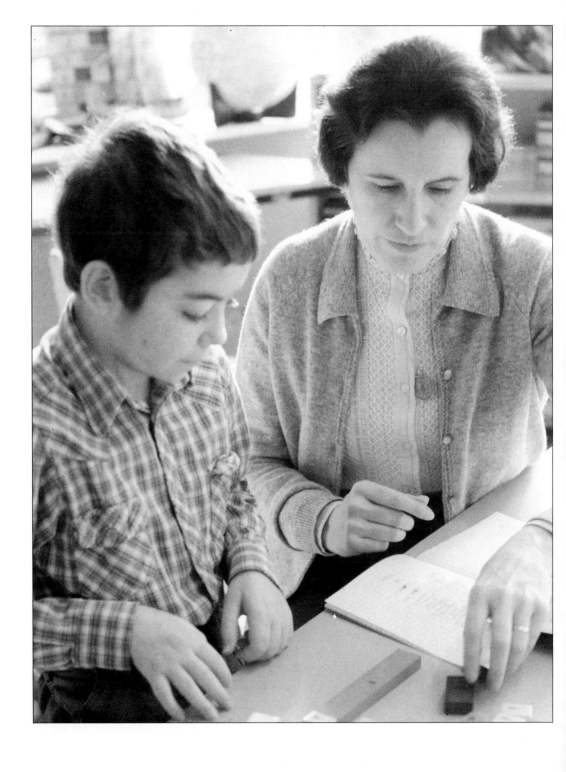

FAMILY HEALTH GUIDE

ARTHRITIS
& RHEUMATISM

LEE RODWELL

WITH THE HELP OF THE
ARTHRITIS AND RHEUMATISM COUNCIL

WARD LOCK

Lee Rodwell
Lee Rodwell is a leading freelance journalist who specialises in health issues, lifestyle and family matters. For the past 10 years, she has been writing for a broad cross-section of the UK magazine and newspaper market. She has written four books and is married with two children.

A WARD LOCK BOOK

First published in the UK 1994
by Ward Lock
Wellington House
125 Strand
London WC2R 0BB
A Cassell Imprint

Reprinted 1995

Designed and produced
by SP Creative Design
147 Kings Road, Bury St Edmunds, Suffolk, England

Editor: Heather Thomas
Art Director: Rolando Ugolini
Illustrations: Peter Orrock and A. Milne (pages 39, 47, 57)

Distributed in the United States
by Sterling Publishing Co., Inc.
387 Park Avenue South, New York, NY 10016-8810

Distributed in Australia
by Capricorn Link(Australia) Pty Ltd
2/13 Carrington Road, Castle Hill, NSW 2154

A British Library Cataloguing in Publication Data
block for this book may be obtained from the British Library.

ISBN 0 7063 7257 3

Printed and bound in Spain

Acknowledgements
The author and publishers would like to thank the Arthritis and Rheumatism Council for all their help and also Professor Paul Dieppe of the University of Bristol Department of Medicine. Our special thanks also go to Greenleaf Communications for their help in researching and providing photographs.
Photographs
Cover photo: Comstock Photo Library
Arthritis and Rheumatism Council: pages 2, 13, 19, 30, 32, 39, 41, 43, 59, 64, 69, 70, 71, 72, 73, 74

Contents

Introduction

As a health writer, I spend many hours talking to people whose lives have been changed by illness of one kind or another. Time and again, they mention how difficult it can be to get the kind of information or support they need.

Certainly, for people who suffer from rheumatism or arthritis – and there are about 20 million in the UK today – information can play a key role in getting the most out of life.

Half the battle in coping with a chronic illness is understanding it; and the other half is getting the practical advice which will help you to learn to live with it from day to day. That is why this book aims to explain the common forms of rheumatic disorders, outline the different kinds of treatment available and suggest a variety of things that you can do to make life easier for yourself both in the home and out and about.

You may not find all the answers you are looking for, but I hope, at least, that you will discover where to go to find them. And I hope, too, that the advice and suggestions in this book will help and encourage you to get on top of your illness rather than letting your illness get the better of you.

Lee Rodwell

Chapter one

What's wrong, doctor?

The different kinds of arthritis and rheumatism

Sooner or later most of us suffer from either rheumatism or arthritis. We may wake up one morning with a stiff neck or frozen shoulder. With the passing of time we may notice the odd twinge in our back or our joints and make rueful remarks about getting older.

If we are lucky we will escape with nothing more than creaky joints which complain from time to time. If we are less fortunate we may have to learn to live with constant pain, struggling to do even the everyday tasks that most people take for granted.

There are more than 200 rheumatic disorders and most of them can affect different people to different degrees. So it is not surprising that people are often confused about what is really meant by the terms rheumatism or arthritis. Part of the problem stems from the way lay people use the terms so loosely – and doctors sometimes fail to make things as clear as they might be.

Yet it can be difficult for a specialist, let alone your family doctor, to make the correct diagnosis straight away. As Paul Dieppe, professor of rheumatology at the Bristol Royal Infirmary in the UK explains: "It is often very difficult to differentiate between early arthritis and muscular aches and pains which may not be of much significance long term.

"The pain may not be very well localized and examinations and tests can be normal in the early stages, so sometimes we have to wait several months and watch people to see what happens until we are sure of a diagnosis. Most aches and pains go away after a while rather than turning into anything serious – and that's why doctors often play a waiting game."

Most people who go to their doctor want the answer to two key questions: What's wrong? Will it get better? The trouble with many common forms of arthritis is that even when doctors have identified the problem, they still cannot predict with any certainty how things will turn out in the long run.

"We know that a certain set of tests and circumstances make it more or less likely that things will get worse long term," says Paul Dieppe, "but although this may help us decide how much treatment we should give early on, statistics don't help when it comes to predicting how a particular patient will fare."

Since every patient is different, your doctor is unlikely to be able to tell you exactly what to expect. That, in itself, can be difficult to cope with. Worse still, you may be unfortunate in dealing with either a doctor or specialist who is not very good at communicating. Because doctors are so familiar with medical terms they sometimes

What's wrong, doctor?

assume everyone knows what they mean. Others try to keep things simple and so you end up with half the story.

This book cannot take the place of a doctor, nor should it. Your doctor is always the first person to go to for help and advice. If you are suffering persistent aches and pains you need to be properly diagnosed and then offered treatment to suit your particular case.

What this book can do is give you information that you can use to help yourself. After all, if you know something about the way your body works and what happens when rheumatic disorders strike, you will be better placed to ask the right questions and take the right course of action.

So let's start at the beginning: what *is* the difference between rheumatism and arthritis?

● **Arthritis** is any disease which attacks the joints, sometimes leaving them damaged.

The word literally means inflammation of the joint, from the Greek *arthron* (joint) and -*itis* (inflammation) but it is used to describe any type of joint disease even when no inflammation is involved.

● **Rheumatism** is a more general term used to cover aches and pains in the bones, muscles, joints and tissues surrounding the joints. So rheumatism includes arthritis. Medical experts prefer to avoid these vaguer terms and talk instead about **rheumatic diseases, rheumatic disorders** or **disorders of the musculoskeletal system.**

Different disorders affect different parts of the musculoskeletal system in different ways. Rheumatoid arthritis, for example, starts in the synovial membrane, whereas in osteoarthritis the joint cartilage is affected first. A brief explanation of how the system works may help you to understand what can go wrong and how best to treat the problem.

The musculoskeletal system

Your body's framework of *bones* is connected up at your *joints*. The joints that move are called the *synovial joints*. These joints include the shoulder, hip, knee and elbow.

● A synovial joint is encased in a joint capsule which is lined with a synovial membrane, or synovium. This contains synovial fluid which lubricates the joint.

Where one bone meets another in a joint capsule, the surface of each is covered by a substance called *articular cartilage*. Synovial fluid is pumped in and out of this as the joint moves or rests.

● Not all of the joints in the body work this way: *fibrous joints* are found where much less movement is needed between the individual bones. A fibrous joint consists of a pad of cartilage between the bones, with no joint cavity. The pad acts like a shock absorber and allows a little movement. The inter-vertebral joints in the spine are fibrous joints.

Joints are connected and moved by soft tissue: muscles, tendons and ligaments. Some muscles are attached directly to the bone; others are attached by tendons. Some tendons run through sliding tunnels lined by

The synovial inflammation of rheumatoid arthritis

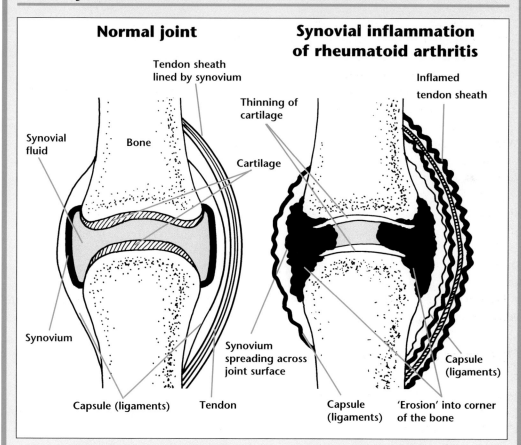

Normal joint

Synovial inflammation of rheumatoid arthritis

Tendon sheath lined by synovium

Thinning of cartilage

Inflamed tendon sheath

Synovial fluid

Bone

Cartilage

Synovium

Synovium spreading across joint surface

Capsule (ligaments)

Capsule (ligaments)

Tendon

Capsule (ligaments)

'Erosion' into corner of the bone

In a normal joint, the synovium layer of tissue secretes synovial fluid, which lubricates and nourishes the cartilage around the bone end. The ligaments help to keep the joint stable. The tendons are attached to the bones and work with the muscles to make the joints move. When a person has rheumatoid arthritis, the synovial tissue, which lines some joints and tendons, becomes inflamed, causing swelling and pain in the joints.

The disease can affect different people in different ways: the number and type of joints affected varies as does the degree of severity and the duration of the inflammation. Some people experience 'flare-ups' in which the inflammation gets worse for a few days or weeks and then subsides.

What's wrong, doctor?

The human skeleton

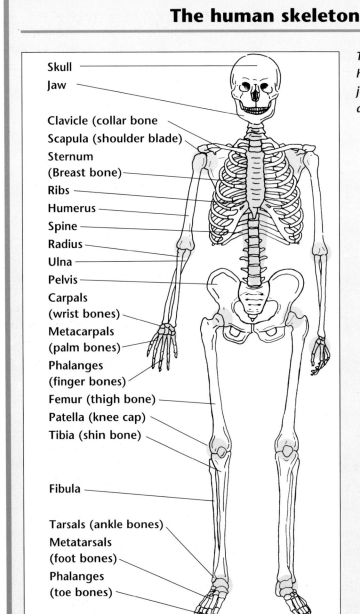

Skull

Jaw

Clavicle (collar bone

Scapula (shoulder blade)

Sternum
(Breast bone)

Ribs

Humerus

Spine

Radius

Ulna

Pelvis

Carpals
(wrist bones)

Metacarpals
(palm bones)

Phalanges
(finger bones)

Femur (thigh bone)

Patella (knee cap)

Tibia (shin bone)

Fibula

Tarsals (ankle bones)

Metatarsals
(foot bones)

Phalanges
(toe bones)

This illustration of the human skeleton shows the joints that are most often affected by arthritis.

the same type of synovial membrane as the joint capsules.

Ligaments also help hold the bones and other parts of the body together. A bursa acts like a protective cushion between a tendon and a bone.

Abnormalities in the body's *immune system* also play a part in many rheumatic disorders. Sometimes, instead of fighting infection and helping the body to restore itself to good health, the immune system attacks the body's own tissues causing damage.

The four categories

Rheumatic disorders

Although there are so many different rheumatic disorders, the World Health Organisation has classified them into four main categories:

1 Back pain.
2 Soft tissue disorders.
3 Osteoarthritis and related disorders.
4 Inflammatory arthritis.

Back pain

Doctors often find it hard to pin-point the cause of back pain even though this is a common problem; more than 75 per cent of all adults suffer from back pain at some time or another.

The spine (or backbone) is made up of small bones called vertebrae. Twenty four of these can move; the seven in the neck (the cervical vertebrae) and the five in the lower back (the lumbar vertebrae) are more mobile than the twelve in the chest (the thoracic vertebrae).

Each vertebra is linked to the next by joints, known as facet joints. At the top of one joint and the bottom of the next is a thin layer of cartilage with a disc in between. The disc not only acts like a cushion, but works rather like a ball bearing, allowing the spine to twist and bend. A complicated network of ligaments holds the spine together, and a range of different muscles controls posture and movement.

The spine is a complicated structure and, like any joint that moves, is subject to wear and tear. However, there are some specific disorders that can cause back pain. These include the following:

Arthritis facts

● There are over 200 forms of arthritic and rheumatic diseases.
● One in 1,000 children suffers from juvenile arthritis.
● Only one in fifty people will escape some form of the disease.
● In the UK, over 6,000,000 people are affected by arthritic and rheumatic diseases.
● Arthritis is the biggest single cause of disability in the UK.

What's wrong, doctor?

Damage to the spine by osteoporosis

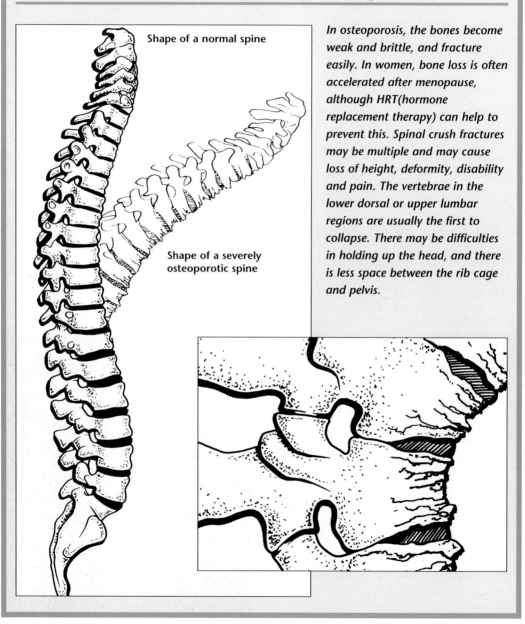

Shape of a normal spine

Shape of a severely osteoporotic spine

In osteoporosis, the bones become weak and brittle, and fracture easily. In women, bone loss is often accelerated after menopause, although HRT(hormone replacement therapy) can help to prevent this. Spinal crush fractures may be multiple and may cause loss of height, deformity, disability and pain. The vertebrae in the lower dorsal or upper lumbar regions are usually the first to collapse. There may be difficulties in holding up the head, and there is less space between the rib cage and pelvis.

● **Prolapsed intervertebral disc** (often called, less accurately, a slipped disc).

● **Ankylosing spondylitis,** an inflammatory arthritis of the spine.

● **Osteoporosis,** a condition in which the bones become weaker and more brittle.

● **Spondylosis,** a degenerative or 'wear and tear' disease in which fringes of bone grow out trapping nerves and stiffening the spine.

Most cases of acute back pain – where the pain comes on suddenly in the neck or lower back, for example – usually clear up completely after a few days or a week or so, without any damage. Some people develop a more long-standing problem, often finding that the pain comes and goes from day to day and week to week.

Although back disorders are a major healthcare problem today, most of them are not associated with any serious disease or arthritis of the spine.

Slipped disc

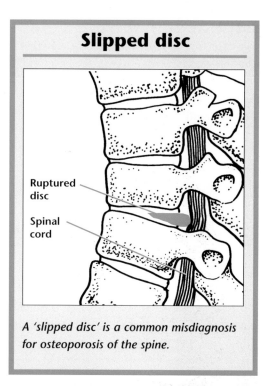

Ruptured disc

Spinal cord

A 'slipped disc' is a common misdiagnosis for osteoporosis of the spine.

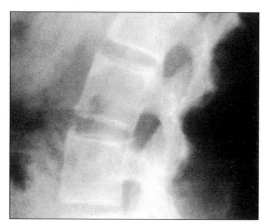

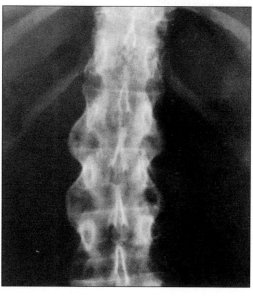

These X-ray pictures show a damaged spine. An X-ray can be used to discover the cause of acute back pain.

What's wrong, doctor?

Soft tissue disorders

Soft tissue (or periarticular) disorders are also widespread. The term covers a whole range of conditions affecting the tissues surrounding a joint. These tissues include muscles, tendons and ligaments.

Most soft tissue disorders are caused by doing an activity we are unaccustomed to, or repeating a particular movement over and over again. Raking up the leaves in the garden once a year may strain the ligaments in your back.

Scrubbing the floor may give you housemaid's knee – otherwise known as bursitis, an inflammation of the bursa.

Over-use injuries can affect a number of the body's tissues. One of the most common complaints is tenosynovitis; this is the inflammation of the tendon sheaths around the wrist or ankle. Sometimes the point where the tendon is attacked to the bone becomes inflamed from repetitive strain; that's why you can get tennis elbow even if you have never played tennis in your life!

Soft tissue disorders may also be caused by injury. You might strain or tear ligaments playing football, or taking part in some other energetic sport.

None of these periarticular disorders is dangerous or causes permanent damage, and treatment is often simple and effective.

However, fibromyalgia, which causes severe pain in the fibrous tissue and muscles as well as overall fatigue, can sometimes be severe and may last for several years.

Tennis elbow

Tennis elbow is caused by physical strain but this may not necessarily be playing too much tennis. People in their forties and fifties are the most affected, and gripping and twisting are very painful. The pain is aggravated by repeated wrist movements, such as using a paint roller on a ceiling, or a backhand tennis stroke. It is very painful but it is not connected to arthritis or any other disease. Refraining from any repetitive movements of the elbow or resting your arm in a sling usually help alleviate the condition. A steroid injection or physiotherapy may be necessary if the pain is severe and lingers.

Osteoarthritis and related disorders

Osteoarthritis is the most common form of joint disease; around five million people in the UK suffer from it. It usually starts when you are in your 50s although it can begin any time after you reach 30. Women are affected a little more often than men and some families are more prone to the condition than others.

At the end of our bones is a thin layer of cartilage which acts as a shock absorber and helps the joint move. The bone end and cartilage are surrounded by a membrane called the synovium.

As the cartilage at the end of the bones wears away, the bone beneath thickens and grows outwards, enlarging the joint. It also forms spurs at the edges of the joint, called osteophytes. These spurs are partly

Fibromyalgia

There are several terms for this condition: fibrositis, non-articular rheumatism and soft-tissue rheumatism. Although it is called 'rheumatism', there is no joint damage and the pain you feel is in the ligaments and muscles.

Fibromyalgia often affects people when they are in their twenties and thirties. It starts with stiffness, swelling, pain and tenderness, often around the knees, elbows, shoulders, neck and the lower spine region.

What causes it?

It is often triggered by an injury or perhaps by a viral infection or by stress. However, there may be no obvious cause and it might just happen without warning. If it occurs as a result of injury, even though the injured part of the body heals and recovers, with fibromyalgia the pain continues and occasionally other areas are affected too.

People often respond to pain and injury by resting the injured part, but if they rest it for too long this may affect the normal recovery process. Your recovery rate may also be influenced by other factors, such as whether you experience stress or severe emotional disturbances at the time of the injury, and your level of physical fitness and how much sleep you get.

Treatment

Your doctor may prescribe medication to relieve the pain or ordinary pain killers such as aspirin, paracetamol and ibuprofen may help, but the most effective treatment rests with you in getting fit and relaxed. Developing your own personal fitness programme will help make you feel healthier and improve your sense of well-being, leading to an improvement in your symptoms. These may even disappear completely, or they may recur occasionally.

Some people find that other forms of physical therapy are helpful, including acupuncture, massage and TENS(transcutaneous electrical nerve stimulation). These may be worth trying, but only in addition to fitness training and relaxation.

In some cases, you may need a local injection if the pain interferes with your normal daily activities, as in the case of tennis or golfer's elbow, bursitis, tendinitis and outer hip or inner knee pain. Steroid treatment may be combined with a local anaesthetic.

Fitness training

In order to get better, it is very important that you are self-disciplined about exercising regularly, getting fit and leading a healthy lifestyle. Talk to your doctor about this and see what he recommends. You may have to start slowly if you are unused to exercise, and build up gradually

continued on page 16

What's wrong, doctor?

continued from page 15
as you get fitter and stronger. This might be uncomfortable and unfamiliar at first, and you may even notice that your symptoms seem to get worse. However, they will improve eventually and it is worth persevering.

Your doctor may recommend that you give up smoking as this adversely affects your ability to exercise as well as threatening your health and increasing the risk of heart disease, bronchitis and lung cancer. You may have to opt for a relatively gentle form of exercise if you suffer from a medical condition such as chronic bronchitis or angina. Walking or using an exercise bike may be suitable in this case. Again, ask your doctor for guidance.

If you dislike exercising alone and find it hard to discipline yourself to do so, you might prefer to exercise with a friend or in a group. You could try swimming, cycling, gentle jogging, or join a keep-fit class. Find out what activities there are in your area.

Planning a fitness programme

Ideally, you should exercise three or four times a week. Don't rush into a fitness regime; take it slowly and only introduce new exercises gradually as you get fitter. You may feel stiff and ache after these sessions in the early days. This is quite normal and will disappear as you get fitter. Warming-up before exercise and cooling-down afterwards will help to prevent this.

A typical fitness programme consists of:
- A warm-up and stretching.
- Aerobic exercises to improve stamina.
- Exercises to improve strength and endurance.
- Circuit training.
- A cool-down and stretching.

This sounds complicated but it isn't really. You could join a gym or go to the fitness suite at your local leisure or sports centre, or you could devise some simple exercises which you can perform at home.

Clothing and equipment

Dress in loose, comfortable clothes which will not restrict your movement, e.g. a tracksuit or leotard and tights. Wear sensible, comfortable shoes such as trainers. You don't need special equipment, although a bench or low stool or table may be useful.

Training and safety rules

- Build up gradually, and don't attempt too much too soon.
- Only stretch as far as feels comfortable.
- If you feel pain, stop at once.
- Listen to your body and what it is telling you; don't try to go too far too fast.
- Always stretch before and after exercising. This will help prevent injuries and reduce stiffness and muscular soreness.

Note: If you are unsure about devising an exercise programme, ask your doctor or physiotherapist for advice.

Osteoarthritic joint

Mild osteoarthritis

Severe osteoarthritis with joint deformity

Thick stretched capsule

Thickened bone growing at side of joint

Inflamed synovium

Thick abnormal bone with no remaining cartilage cover

Loss of remaining cartilage

Mild inflammatory reaction in synovium

Thin damaged cartilage with uneven surface and 'splits' in the surface

Distorted damaged capsule

In osteoarthritis, the surface of the joint is damaged and there is an abnormal reaction in the underlying bone. The cartilage becomes thinner with a rougher surface; the bone underneath becomes thicker and grows out at the side of the joint. In severe cases, the cartilage may be damaged so badly that the bone is exposed and the joint may become deformed.

responsible for the gnarled appearance of the hands you sometimes see in older people with the disorder.

The synovium may become inflamed and the extra fluid that forms may make the joint swell slightly, becoming stiff and painful.

There are many different types of osteoarthritis affecting different joints. The most commonly affected joints are the knees, hands, hips and big toes.

Osteoarthritis tends to creep up on you over the years but it does not always go on getting worse and worse. Even people who are quite severely affected often find that bad spells are interspersed with periods where they are much better.

Many people are so mildly affected that they never have to seek medical help. However, some sufferers do have severe joint damage, pain and disability.

What's wrong, doctor?

Inflammatory arthritis

This group of disorders includes some of the most severe, painful and disabling diseases which may begin as early as childhood. As the name suggests, inflammation causes painful swelling of the joints which may feel hot and look red. The different types of inflammatory arthritis include the following conditions.

Rheumatoid arthritis (RA)

Although rheumatoid arthritis can affect anyone at any age, women are three times more likely than men to suffer from it. No one knows what causes the disease although research suggests there may be a number of factors that trigger it. One may be a viral or bacterial infection. Another may be your genetic make-up: even though you cannot inherit the disease something in your genes may make you more likely to contract it.

Once the process has been triggered the body's immune system over-reacts, attacking the body's own joint tissues. Instead of getting better, the inflammation persists.

The effects of RA

RA affects different people in different ways. Sometimes only one or two joints are affected. In other cases the disease is widespread and very active. About 30 per cent of people who contract RA appear to recover completely within a few years. About 65 per cent continue to suffer pains in their joints, swellings and sudden flare-ups, while around five per cent become severely affected and extensively disabled.

Juvenile chronic arthritis

Most people tend to assume that arthritis is something which only affects the elderly but there are several types which may occur in childhood.

Most children who develop juvenile arthritis early in life go on to make a good recovery. Some forms of childhood arthritis clear up quickly; in other cases families have to work closely with their doctors and physiotherapists to make sure that as little permanent damage is done to their child's joints as possible. Children with arthritis often need to wear splints and follow a regular exercise programme. Sometimes surgery is necessary.

Ankylosing spondylitis (AS)

The third most common rheumatic disorder, this affects more men than women. Also known as 'poker back' because of the effect it can have on the patient, it begins with inflammation at the entheses. This is the place where the ligaments and tendons are attached to the bones in the spine.

The bone responds by growing out from both sides of the joint and can end up surrounding it completely, fusing one vertebra to the next. AS sometimes affects other joints, such as the hips, knees, ankles or shoulders.

Psoriatic arthritis

As the name suggests, this form of inflammatory arthritis sometimes affects people with psoriasis. Although it is a similar condition to rheumatoid arthritis, it is generally milder in its effects.

It does not necessarily develop where the skin is affected with the characteristic red, scaly patches but most commonly strikes the spine, knees or hands. Often the person's fingernails become pitted and discoloured.

Gout

Despite the myths, gout is not the result of a lifetime of heavy drinking, although alcohol can exacerbate the condition. Gout occurs when the body's system for disposing of excess uric acid fails and uric acid builds up in the blood. Eventually uric acid crystals form in the joints causing pain, redness and swelling.

Gout often manifests itself in the big toe joints, although the knees, elbows and wrists may also be affected.

Lupus

Systemic lupus erythematosus, to give it its full name, is a connective tissue disorder which often affects the joints, causing arthritis. However, many of the body's organs and tissues may be involved.

Lupus can be very difficult to diagnose because the symptoms and extent of the disorder can vary so much from one person to another.

Whatever your problem, it is worth remembering that doctors now know a great deal more about rheumatic diseases than they did in the past – and they are learning more all the time. Even if your doctor cannot give you all the answers you are looking for,

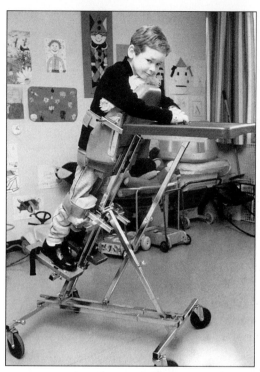

Arthritis is not just an adult disease; it affects children, too. About one in a thousand children are affected by chronic(persistent) arthritis in the early years of their lives. It is not known what causes the disease in children, but it usually starts between the ages of one and four years, and can occur at any time throughout childhood.

he can offer the prospect of treatment that will help. As the British Arthritis and Rheumatism Research Council says: 'Advances in treatment, therapy and joint replacement have been significant. There is no need for most rheumatic patients to suffer unduly or have their lives unnecessarily restricted by the disease.'

What's wrong, doctor?

The areas affected most by inflammatory arthritis

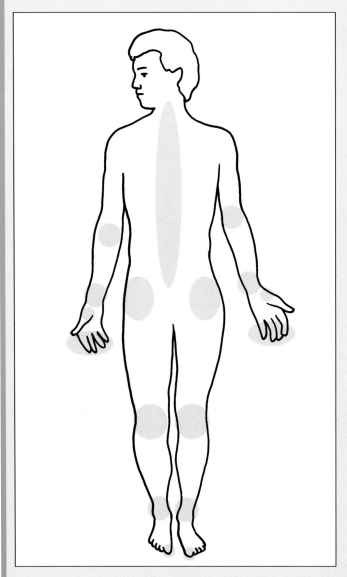

This artwork illustration shows the parts of the body that are most affected by inflammatory arthritis, including the neck, lower back and hips, knees, base of thumb and ends of fingers. The joints swell painfully and may become hot and red as a result of the inflammation. There are several types of this sort of arthritis, the best known of which is rheumatoid arthritis which can affect anyone at any age.

Gout

Men of any age can be affected by gout, the most easily treated form of rheumatic disease. Women are less affected and then only after menopause. Gout runs in families and is usually inherited. We all have uric acid in our blood but sometimes something goes wrong with the chemical processes in our body, and instead of the excess uric acid being passed into the urine, it is deposited in the joints and forms crystals, making the joints very painful.

These crystals may also appear under the skin like little white pimples(tophi), especially on the ear lobes and hands. The uric acid may also be deposited in the body's internal organs, especially the kidneys.

Even if the body's uric acid level is high, it may not necessarily lead to gout. However, if you do suffer an attack of gout, it is extremely painful. The pain usually starts in the big toe, which becomes red, swollen and tender. Other joints may also be attacked, notably the knees, elbows and wrists.

If you are prone to gout, it can be triggered off as a result of:
- An injury or bruising to a joint.
- Fatigue, worry or illness.
- An operation.
- Excessive eating and drinking.
- Anything which upsets your system.

Watch out for the early warning signs of an attack of gout so that you can start treatment before it gets worse. The first few attacks will not damage your joints permanently and you will recover. In mild cases, there may even be years between attacks. However, more rarely, if you suffer persistent attacks of gout, the joint can eventually become damaged by the uric acid crystals and trigger off chronic arthritis.

Diagnosis of gout

Gout may be diagnosed by the following means:
- A blood test to measure the amount of uric acid in the blood.
- X-rays of joints.
- Examining joint fluid.

Treatment of gout

Regular preventive treatment may be necessary to control levels of uric acid in the body. Your doctor may prescribe tablets to help maintain normal blood levels of urate. The most common drug is allopurinol and this is very safe, even when taken for years, the only possible side effect being a rash. Remember that preventive treatment usually means life-time treatment.

Acute attacks are usually treated with non-steroidal anti-inflammatory analgesics(NSAIDS), which help relieve pain and inflammation. They have little effect on uric acid levels in the blood nor do they prevent further attacks. Side effects are rare, but occasionally a patient with an allergy may suffer indigestion, a rash, headache, dizziness or even asthma.

Chapter two

From drugs to surgery

Treatments your doctor may suggest

The treatment your doctor or specialist will suggest will depend on a variety of factors, not least the kind of disorder you have and the extent to which this is causing you pain or disrupting your life.

You might be prescribed one of a number of different drugs. Surgery may be necessary. Perhaps you will be sent to see a physiotherapist who will help suggest some exercises to keep you mobile.

Surgery

For people who suffer a great deal from rheumatoid arthritis or osteoarthritis, surgery can make a big difference to the quality of their lives. Who else may be offered it?

Some people with ankylosing spondylitis may occasionally need surgery on their spine or hips and a small number of those with other, less common, forms of joint disease may also need an operation. But most people with milder forms of rheumatism or arthritis will never need surgery at all.

The operations, like the diseases, are of two main kinds: those outside the joint (periarticular) and those on the joint proper (articular).

Periarticular surgery, which includes repairing damaged ligaments and tendons and removing large cysts and nodules, is generally relatively minor.

Articular surgery falls into four different categories, of which joint replacement is probably the one we have all heard about.

Joint replacement

Most people have something read about hip replacement operations, but knee replacements are now almost as reliable and as commonplace. Joint replacement for the shoulders and elbows is also progressing and it is also possible to replace the small joints of the hand and ankle.

All of this is thanks to the development of modern metal alloy and high density plastics, but artificial joints are not perfect. They don't last for ever, they don't function as well as a natural joint, and in about one case in twenty the operation is not a complete success.

Joint replacements

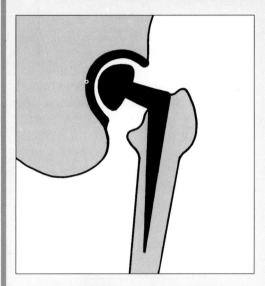

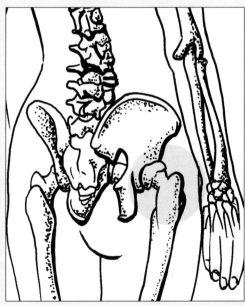

Hip replacement is the most common operation, but it will not be suggested by your doctor or specialist unless you have severe pain and until every other possibility has been investigated. Your specialist will choose the best artificial joint for you.

Complications are very rare and every possible care is taken to prevent them. However, infection can occur around the artificial joint in one to two per cent of patients. This can be treated effectively with antibiotics.

Artificial hip joints seldom wear out and they will last for years. You can walk, drive your car, cycle, dance and play golf – in short, lead a normal life. Very energetic sports are not recommended, e.g. tennis, but if you play them gently they are probably all right. You may not be able to bend your leg upwards as far as you would like, especially in the first six to eight weeks after the operation.

You will have to get used to walking with your new hip and may need sticks at first. The time to recover and get back to work varies. Some people recover enough to go back to work after six weeks; others take six months.

From drugs to surgery

Synovectomy

If the lining of the joint is very bulky and inflamed it may not only stop the joint from moving but may also threaten to damage the ligaments or tendons. Under these circumstances it may be necessary to operate to remove the joint lining.

Arthrosis

This operation is sometimes used when a joint is already restricted but is still very painful. The surgeon will fix the joint permanently, either by bone grafting or by nailing or wiring the two halves together. Afterwards, the joint can no longer move, but it is no longer painful.

Osteotomy

Osteotomy involves cutting the bone next to a painful joint and then refixing it in a slightly different position. It can correct a deformity and relieve the pain of osteoarthritis, mostly in the knee or foot. It can also stimulate healing of the joint.

Most joints can be operated on, but only a few procedures are commonly used Hand surgery can be carried out to repair tendons and release trapped nerves. People who suffer badly from rheumatoid arthritis may be offered operations on their feet, to cut out the damaged joints at the base of their toes so that they can walk without pain. Bunion operations are also common.

What can you do

If your specialist suggests surgery, check out all the pros and cons before deciding to go ahead. It is always a good idea to take along a list of questions you want to ask and to jot down the answers you are given.

Don't forget to ask about the details; how long will you be in hospital, how long will you be in plaster, what will you be able to do a week, a month, a year after the operation?

Ask about the possibilities of any complications and try to be realistic about the benefits you will gain. When it comes to surgery, there are no guarantees.

Try to talk to others who have had a similar operation, bearing in mind that no two people are ever the same.

Is surgery necessary?

If your doctor rules out surgery, ask him why. Sometimes surgeons will be reluctant to operate because of your age. Although hip replacements, for instance, have been very successful for the elderly, the results have not been so good in younger adults.

As Professor Dieppe says: "One of the most difficult tasks for doctors is to recommend the right operation at the right time."

Drug treatments

Although there are no drugs that can cure rheumatism or arthritis there are a number of drug treatments that can help. Drugs often make the difference between being able to get out and about or being stuck at home. Different treatments work differently for different people, so it may take a while for your doctor to discover what is the most effective regime for you.

Drugs can also cause side effects and, again, these may differ from one person to the next. Drugs may react with each other, so if you are taking any other medication (even over-the-counter remedies), it is important that your doctor knows about this. Different drugs need to be taken at different times and in different ways; some should be taken before eating, for instance.

Drug treatment

There are two main types of drug used to treat rheumatoid arthritis: anti-inflammatory drugs and anti-rheumatoid drugs. Simple pain killers are also used as are steroids but more rarely.

Anti-inflammatory drugs
These drugs treat the symptoms rather than the disease itself; they reduce pain, swelling and stiffness. Aspirin is the best known of these, but high doses can upset the stomach and cause indigestion.

Anti-rheumatoid drugs
These drugs are remission inducing. Not only do they help alleviate the symptoms but they also help prevent the condition getting progressively worse. Some people respond so well to treatment that they get almost complete remission from rheumatoid arthritis, whereas others experience more modest results. They act

more slowly than anti-inflammatory drugs, often taking months to produce benefits. The most common of these drugs are: sulphasalazine, chloroquine and hydroxychloroquine, gold and D-penicillamine.

Immunosuppressive drugs
These are sometimes used in treating rheumatoid arthritis. They work by affecting the body's immune system. However, although effective, they can cause anaemia.

Steroids and cortisone-like drugs
Generally, these are used only in special circumstances. Steroid injections into the affected joints can bring short-term pain relief and reduction of inflammation, but they cannot be given too often. Steroid tablets are sometimes prescribed, usually in small doses.

From drugs to surgery

For all these reasons, it is a good idea to keep your own medical diary. If you take the diary with you when you go to visit your doctor or specialist you can make a note of the name of the drug you are prescribed, what it aims to do for you, and when and how you should take it.

You can also note what side-effects to watch out for, and you can record these if and when they occur. Keep a note, too, of what the doctor says about stopping the drug altogether or reducing the dosage, and what you should do if you miss a dose for any reason.

Most of us can recall coming out of the doctor's surgery and finding ourselves unable

Medicine containers

Remember, too, to tell the pharmacist if you cannot open the child-proof containers in which most drugs are dispensed. He will be able to give you an alternative.

to recall everything we have been told, but if you make a note at the time you will avoid this. And don't forget that the pharmacist can also answer most of the questions you might have if you do happen to remember something you wish you had asked.

What kind of drugs are used?

Drug treatments

There are four main types of drugs used in the treatment of rheumatic disorders.

1 Pain killers.
2 Anti-inflammatory drugs.
3 Steroids.
4 Drugs that control or modify specific diseases.

Pain killers

Despite their name, pain killers do not 'kill' pain and do nothing to treat the underlying cause of the discomfort. A better name for them might be pain dullers. They work by interfering with the process by which the body sends out pain signals which are then received by the brain. Some block the transmission of these signals on the way to the brain, whereas others work on the brain itself so that it ignores the signals it receives. Pain killers may sometimes have side effects: for instyance, they can cause drowsiness and some may cause constipation.

Simple mild pain killers, such as aspirin, paracetamol and codeine, can be bought over the counter at the pharmacy without a prescription. Sometimes doctors will prescribe slightly stronger ones such as dextropropoxyphene, but the really strong, addictive drugs, such as pethidine and morphine, are hardly ever used.

Sometimes mixtures of small doses of two or three pain killers seem to work better than one on its own, but you must be careful not to exceed the recommended doses. If you are going to take a mixture of pain killers, you must talk to your doctor first.

Most pain killers work only for a few hours. The sensible way to use them is to limit yourself to times when the pain is particularly bad, or to take a dose just before doing something you know from experience will be painful. However, some people who are severely affected by arthritis do need regular pain killers in addition to other treatments.

Anti-inflammatory agents

Anti-inflammatory agents (non steroidal anti-inflammatory drugs or NSAIDS) Since these drugs reduce inflammation they also reduce pain, swelling and stiffness. So if you have rheumatoid arthritis, rather than osteoarthritis, they may be much better at relieving pain than ordinary pain killers.

However, NSAIDS can cause indigestion and, sometimes, ulcers. Other uncommon side effects can include drowsiness, rashes and fluid retention.

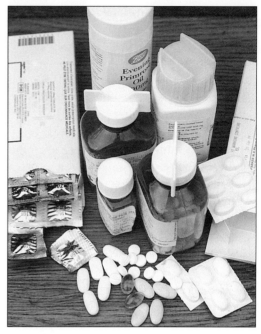

Taken in high doses, aspirin can reduce inflammation but it can irritate the stomach. Excessive use may also cause tinnitus (ringing in the ears). Modern NSAIDS are safer and are less likely to cause side-effects.

A whole range of these drugs is now

NSAIDS and gastric trouble

Since NSAIDS relieve pain, a peptic ulcer (or even, in rare cases, a perforated stomach or duodenum) may seem to appear out of the blue. How can you try to prevent any problems?.

● Always take the NSAID with, or else immediately after, food, never on an empty stomach.

● Tell your doctor if you have any indigestion pain.
● Keep an eye on your bowel motions. If they are black or dark grey this may suggest gastric bleeding.
● If you have severe stomach pains see your doctor at once or go straight to a hospital.

available. Indomethacin (Indocid) is one of the most widely prescribed. Others include naproxen (Naprosyn), diclofenac sodium (Voltarol) and ibuprofen (Brufen or Nurofen). NSAIDS come in a variety of forms including tablets, capsules, syrups and suppositories.

Many people need a period of trial and error to see which of these drugs works best for them. You should try each drug for two weeks to see if there are any benefits. Sometimes a dose taken at night is enough to reduce stiffness and pain in the mornings.

If you have been taking a drug for a while and you are not sure whether it is doing any good you can always try going without for a week to see if there is any difference. After all, there is no point going on taking a drug if it isn't helping.

Steroids

Steroids are hormones that occur naturally in the body. They control the body's metabolism in a variety of ways and their main value in treating arthritis is to reduce inflammation and damp down the body's defence system. They can be given in tablet form or by injection into a joint which is particularly inflamed or painful, or by intramuscular or intravenous injection ('pulse therapy').

Drug dependence

If you take high doses for a long time it is possible to become addicted; then it is dangerous to reduce the dose too quickly.

Adverse reactions of NSAIDS

The major adverse drug reactions of NSAIDS are listed below:
- Gastrointestinal: indigestion, nausea, peptic ulceration, gastric erosion.
- Renal: fluid retention, hypertension, renal impairment.
- Skin: photosensitivity.
- Haematological: iron deficiency anaemia.
- Central effects: headaches, dizziness, confusion.

In some disorders steroids are essential to prevent serious problems. Even so, they need to be carefully controlled and in other cases they are better used sparingly or in low doses to get things under control. Used over a long period they can cause a variety of side-effects including thinning of bones and skin, cataracts, fluid retention and raised blood pressure.

Drugs that modify disease

These drugs not only help relieve symptoms, but also seem to slow down a disease or prevent permanent damage. Some people respond so well that the disease practically goes away; others experience only a slight improvement. It often takes weeks or even months for these drugs to start producing benefits.

Most of these drugs can cause side effects and so you need to be monitored carefully, although the drugs for gout are very safe. Gout patients cannot take aspirin as this raises the levels of uric acid in the blood. Instead they are likely to be prescribed allopurinol (which stops too much uric acid forming) or a drug such as probenecid which helps the kidneys get rid of uric acid. Since these drugs aim to prevent further attacks, a sufferer may also be given an anti-inflammatory drug or colchicine as well for the first few weeks.

The commonly used disease-modifying drugs for other inflammatory joint diseases fall into two categories: the drugs that suppress the body's immune system and a miscellaneous group.

The first group includes azathioprine and cyclophosphamide. These powerful drugs are sometimes used in treating rheumatoid arthritis. Patients need to have regular blood tests to make sure that the drugs are not causing anaemia or other problems.

The second group includes gold injections, D-penicillamine, chloroquine, hydroxychloroquine, methotrexate and sulphasalazine.

● **Gold injections** have been used to treat RA since the 1920s, although methods have now changed. Providing the proper precautions are taken, this treatment is very safe. Some doctors now use a new type of gold in tablet form.

● **D-penicillamine** can be taken even by people who are allergic to its distant relative, penicillin. Patients begin with a small dose which is built up gradually over a few months.

● **Chloroquine and hydroxychloroquine** are generally used to treat and prevent malaria but they also have an anti-rheumatoid effect. However, a high dose given over a long period may affect the eyes, so patients may need regular eye-checks to prevent this.

● **Suphasalazine** has been in common use for the past ten years. It is taken by mouth and the dose is increased over a few weeks. Some patients feel sick when they start to take it, but this is generally a temporary side effect.

● **Methotrexate** has become very popular for the treatment of many forms of arthritis. It is a slow acting but effective anti-inflammatory agent which also slows down disease progression. It is usually given as tablets, once a week. It can occasionally damage the liver or lungs, but is generally very safe if used in the way instructed.

Drugs and you

Although there is now a wide range of drugs that can be used to help people with rheumatism and arthritis they should all be used carefully and under regular supervision.

The more information you have, the more you can discuss your own case with your doctor. It's important for you to know what kind of drugs you are being offered and why.

And it is up to you to take responsibility for following instructions and keeping a record of how the drugs are affecting you.

From drugs to surgery

The future

Scientists are now working on a new generation of drugs they call 'the biologics'. These aim to target the mechanisms in the pathways that cause rheumatic disease. Some of these drugs are on trial now, and researchers are very excited about the possibilities of treating many common rheumatic diseases, and particularly rheumatoid arthritis.

However, a great deal of work still needs to be done and it will be many years yet before these drugs become widely available, although they do hold out new hope for arthritis suffers in the future.

Therapy

A number of different therapists may be able to help you reduce the pain and stay mobile.

Physiotherapists are trained to treat disorders of the musculoskeletal system and can use a variety of techniques to help you get your body to function better. These techniques include special exercises (which you can be taught to do at home), and manipulation and hydrotherapy. A physiotherapist may use heat or ice packs to

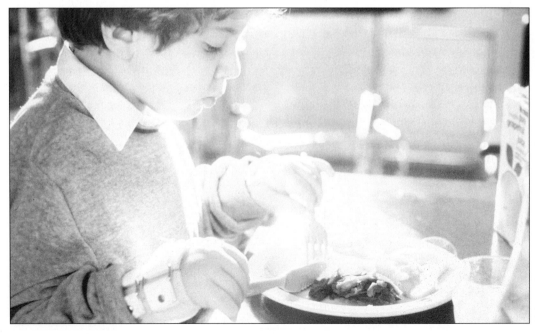

Footwear

Special footwear and orthotics may sometimes be prescribed for rheumatoid arthritis sufferers. If this happens to you, it is important that you wear the device or the whole process has failed. Even if you do not need special shoes, you should take care when choosing footwear and opt for comfort rather than high fashion.

Choosing shoes
● There should be at least 1cm/½ inch of room at the front of the big toe.
● Your foot should not be able to slide about within the shoe.
● The soles should be light and pliable and capable of bending along an imaginary line drawn from the base of the little toe to the joint at the base of the big toe.
● Leather is most comfortable if you have foot problems.
● Suede finishes and dark colours help disguise mis-shapen feet.
● A heel counter will stop your foot sliding backwards, and lace-up shoes prevent the foot sliding forwards.
● Walking is more comfortable with a low heel.

To check shoe length
Check that a shoe is the right length for you by placing your foot lengthways on a strip of flexible card(1cm/½ inch wide). Mark where your heel and longest toe come, and cut the strip to this measure.

When you are buying shoes, place the strip inside the shoe with one end flush to the heel. If the shoe length is right for you, you should be able to slide the card forwards at least 1cm/½ inch.

Bunions
These are caused by tight, ill-fitting shoes, or by court-style shoes in which the foot is prevented from sliding forwards only by the wedging effect of the toe box. The toes are compressed and bunions may form if the shoes are too pointed or short.

Special problems for arthritis sufferers
● In early rheumatoid arthritis, some women manage by wearing sandals in the summer and fur-lined boots in the winter.
● Shoes can be made specially in soft leather using a plaster-of-Paris replica of your feet.
● For really bad feet, disposable foam plastic shoes can be supplied, padded or cut to fit any shape of foot.
● Laces can be a problem if you have arthritic fingers. Use elastic ones or choose shoes with a Velcro flap. Zip-sided boots are another alternative.
● If you suffer from hallux rigidus, a condition in which the big toe is stiff and won't bend upwards, you can get the sole of your shoe modified.
● If you have stiff ankles and can't point your toes, you need the right heel height and laces right down to the toes.

From drugs to surgery

soothe the pain, or an ultrasound machine to encourage muscles, ligaments or tendons to heal after being injured.

Occupational therapists can help you cope at home and when you are out and about. They can show you ways of adapting your day-to-day life so that you can stay independent, and can give advice on reducing stress, both physical and mental.

Orthotists and chiropodists may also play a useful part in keeping you active. Orthotists make splints which rest inflamed joints and support unstable ones. They can give advice on walking aids and special shoes. Chiropodists can help treat painful corns and bunions and advise on foot care.

Splints

Splints are sometimes prescribed by rheumatologists for the following reasons:
- To rest inflamed joints: to prevent movement and support joints.
- To help increase function in a limb.

Resting splints
These are often used, especially at night, to rest and immobilize joints. For example, they are often used to immobilize the wrist and hand joints of a person with rheumatoid arthritis.

Working splints
Unlike resting splints, these allow a limb to move in a functional way and may include a moving part.

Functions of splints
- To reduce pain and inflammation.
- To stabilize joints.
- To protect joints.
- To prevent or reduce deformity.
- To allow a limb to work in a functional way.

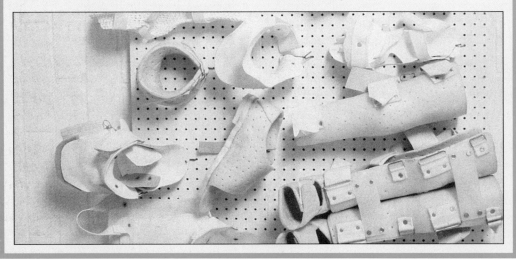

Chapter three

Not what the doctor ordered

Alternative therapies

Given that rheumatism and arthritis are so common, it is not surprising that all kinds of alternative methods of treatment have grown up over the years. People will try almost anything if it promises relief from pain and the hope of a fuller life; and, human nature being what it is, there are always those who are keen to make money out of their desperation.

So how can you tell what holds out a genuine chance of success, or what is likely to be a complete waste of time and money? The chances are that your doctor will be less than enthusiastic about many of the alternative treatments on offer. He probably thinks, with some justification, that if all these things worked, his waiting room would no longer be full of patients, some of them, no doubt, wearing copper bracelets which cannot have anything other than a placebo effect!

However, there are some things you can try that doctors are still keeping an open mind about, and others which, even if they are unlikely to do you any good, at least will not do you any harm and may even help make you feel better.

Diet

Some people swear that changing their diet has made a huge difference to their lives, and the whole debate about whether or not there are links between what you eat and the way you feel has been gathering momentum in recent years.

There are now a number of books which are devoted to arthritis and diet, all of them recommending different regimes. Although doctors tend to feel that experimenting with your diet will make little difference, they are more prepared these days to suspend their scepticism, providing you are not going to restrict yourself so much that you put your health at risk.

One of the problems is that we have very little scientific evidence to show that diet does make a difference, although there are plenty of arthritis sufferers who will give you chapter and verse on how their diet works for them.

Although we know that a change of diet

Not what the doctor ordered

can help improve certain types of arthritis in animals, the same kind of proof is not available when it comes to humans. This is partly because there are so many different types of arthritis, and partly because the common forms vary so much from one person to the next. Besides, most people tend to have good and bad patches, so that it makes it hard to tell whether any improvement in their condition is down to a change in diet, or whether it would have happened anyway.

In addition, you have to take the placebo effect into consideration. In other words, if you believe something is going to work, then it may help you feel better just because you expect it to do so.

Many people want to do something to help themselves. Changing your diet is a fairly easy thing to do and may make you feel better about yourself simply because it gives you a feeling of having some kind of control.

On the other hand, you could end up feeling depressed or disappointed if, after all your efforts, you reap little reward. So what kind of changes do people make?

The 'Eskimo' diet

Many claims have been made about the healthy effect of fish oils. It is true that Eskimos who have always eaten plenty of oily fish have had low rates of heart disease, but can fish oil supplements help curb inflammation and also ease the pain in your joints?

Cold water fish, such as mackerel, salmon and cod, contain oils that are high in polyun-

Trigger foods

Some people feel that certain foods trigger off attacks of pain and swelling in their joints. If they learn to identify and avoid these foods their condition improves.

Different people say that different foods act as triggers: for example, cheese, citrus fruits, dairy products and food colourings. Sometimes people go on an *exclusion diet*, where they cut out groups of foods altogether to see if any might be causing particular problems. If you are interested in this kind of approach there are several things to remember:
● It's advisable to check with your doctor first. If you cut out some foods you may not be getting all the nutrients your body needs and will have to make up the balance in another way.
● You need to be prepared to keep a diary, charting your food intake and noting the results – and you need to be strong willed enough to resist temptation!
● If your condition seems to improve you should double-check the elimination effect by reintroducing the foods you cut out, one at a time. Only then, if the symptoms return, do you need to choose whether you want to avoid these foods altogether.

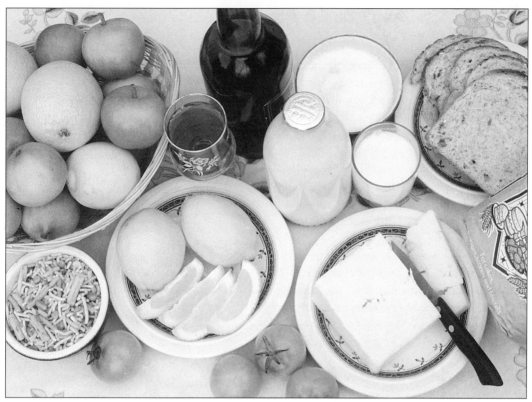

saturated fats, or PUFAS. Sunflower oil and evening primrose oil also contain these PUFAS.

Studies have shown that these fatty acids are used by the body to make chemicals which are less inflammatory than those made from fats in a normal diet. So eating oily fish, or taking fish oil or evening primrose oil supplements, may have an anti-inflammatory effect.

Some people have found that reducing the amount of saturated fat in the diet and taking extra fish or vegetable oils have not only relieved some of their symptoms, but also enabled them to reduce the number of pain killers they need.

Many people claim that certain specific foods can trigger swelling and pain in their joints, especially milk, cheese and dairy products, citrus fruit(oranges, lemons etc.) and some food colourings. However, there is no scientific evidence of this.

The approved medical line is that this kind of diet is unlikely to help most sufferers – but it could help some and it probably won't do anyone any harm. However, anyone with a blood disorder or bleeding problems should only take fish oil under strict medical supervision. Ask your doctor for his views.

Not what the doctor ordered

Other supplements and remedies

● **Selenium** is one of the trace elements, so called because our bodies need only a trace to keep us healthy. There is some evidence that selenium and zinc play a part in the way our immune system works and so, the argument runs, selenium could help in treating arthritis. Once again, however, there is no real evidence that taking extra selenium (with vitamins A, C and E, as is usually suggested) will make any difference.

● **Green-lipped mussel extract** is another supplement that some people claim has anti-inflammatory properties. There is no hard and fast evidence to prove that taking this supplement will be of any benefit, and people allergic to sea-food should steer well clear.

● **Calcium** is needed by children and adults to build strong bones. If you have rheumatoid arthritis – particularly if you are being treated with high doses of steroids – you should make sure that you are getting enough of this important mineral.

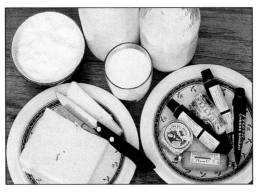

Gout

Gout is the one form of arthritis where diet definitely plays a part. People with gout tend to have higher levels of uric acid than normal and these levels can be affected by food and alcohol. Being overweight increases the production of uric acid. The most important dietary thing to do is to lose some weight if you have gout and are overweight.

Foods with high levels of purines (protein food particles) should only be eaten in moderation or avoided altogether. Examples of such foods include yeast extract, bacon, cod and sardines. Beer is also high in purines because it contains yeast. Your doctor should give you a diet advice sheet.

Supplements can be useful if you don't drink much milk or eat dairy products, such as cheese and yogurt.

● **Herbal remedies** are now widely available in health shops and chemists. Many people think they must be safer than prescribed drugs or medicines because they are 'natural', but they are just as likely to cause side-effects and most will not have been as stringently tested for safety. Check with your doctor before you try any of them. Apart from anything else, they may interfere with any medicines prescribed for you.

Watching your weight

One thing we do know about diet and arthritis is that eating too much of anything is not a good idea: there are definite links between being overweight and developing osteoarthritis of the knees, and gout. Conversely, if you already have arthritis, losing weight will reduce the load on those painful joints.

The less you weigh, the more mobile you will be, and the more exercise you will be able to take. That will burn off more calories.

If you need to lose weight, don't go on a diet, at least, not one of those 'lose 7 pounds in 7 days' kind. Research has shown that when people cut out all their favourite foods at once, or try to restrict their eating unreasonably, they are doomed to failure.

The more deprived you feel, the more likely you are to give in to temptation. The chances are you will then feel guilty and eat to cheer yourself up.

● Do not skip meals, but eat regularly so that you avoid the temptation to snack in between.

● If you do get hungry between meals, eat fruit or even a slice of toast rather than biscuits, cakes, sweets or crisps, and other fatty or sugary snacks.

● Make starchy foods, such as rice, potatoes and pasta, the main part of most meals. These are filling rather than fattening. Add plenty of fresh fruit and vegetables.

● Watch your intake of sugars and fats, especially where these are 'hidden' in processed foods. Avoid fried foods – grill or steam them instead.

Homeopathy

Homeopathy aims to help the body heal itself. Based on the principle that 'like cures like', a homeopathic remedy uses a minute amount of a substance to treat the very condition it would cause if given in greater amounts. For instance, Rhus tox, the American poison ivy, *causes* stiff joints in the morning in healthy people. However, homeopaths use it to *relieve* stiff joints.

The amounts used in homeopathic remedies are so tiny that sceptics feel that they cannot possibly have any effect at all. However, others say the benefits they experience cannot be put down entirely to the placebo effect.

You can buy homeopathic remedies in tablet form at many chemists. Some of those suggested for rheumatism and arthritis include apis mel, arnica, bryonia and rhus tox. You can also get rhus tox and arnica creams to rub into painful joints and muscles.

You may be surprised to learn that many homeopaths are also qualified doctors. All homeopaths will take a full history of the patient's illness and will choose a remedy based on the individual's personality and

Not what the doctor ordered

lifestyle as well as their symptoms. The advantage of seeing a medically qualified homeopath is that they are trained in diagnosis, can also prescribe conventional drugs if appropriate, and will see homeopathy as something to be used as well as, rather than instead of, conventional treatment.

Osteopathy, chiropractic, manipulation

Any treatment that uses stretching, massage or manipulation must be approached with caution. For some people, those with back pain, for example, this kind of approach may give relief when all else has failed. On the other hand, as the Arthritis and Rheumatism Council points out: "Given to the wrong patient or in the wrong way it can be disastrous, particularly when applied to the neck."

It is important to check with your doctor before having treatment and you should not have any kind of manipulation if your condition has flared up again or if you are suffering any inflammation.

If you do consult an osteopath or a chiropractor make sure that they are properly qualified. In the UK, the General Council and Register of Osteopaths and the British Chiropractic Association can give you lists of practitioners. Most of these are in private practice and you will have to pay for their services.

Physiotherapy

Don't forget that physiotherapists are also trained in massage and manipulation. Your doctor can refer you to a physiotherapy department at a local hospital or to an individual therapist.

Spiritual healing

As is the case with so many alternative therapies, there is no independent scientific evidence to show that spiritual healing really works.

It is worth noting that responsible healers do not offer 'miracle cures' Many see themselves as a conduit for some form of external energy which then stimulates the patient's own healing powers. Some patients say that whereas spiritual healing does not actually 'heal' them, it gives them the inner strength to cope better with their physical problems.

Even if the joints in your hands are badly swollen, you can still enjoy many crafts and hobbies. Keeping your fingers mobile by performing the exercises suggested by your doctor and physiotherapist will be helpful.

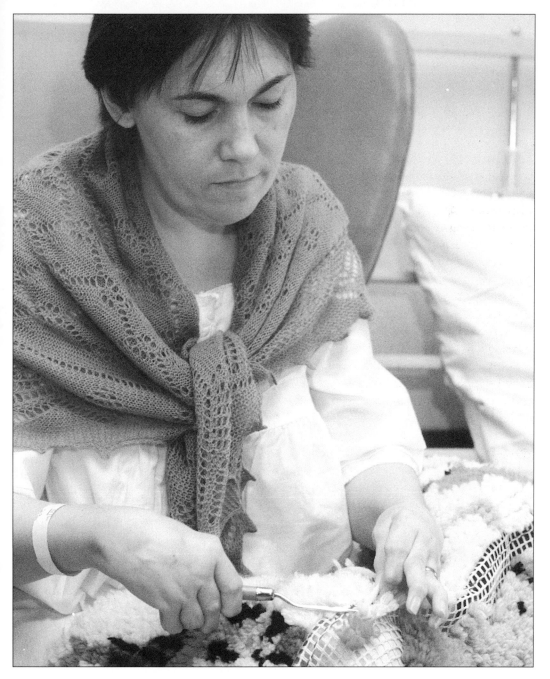

Chapter four

Taking control

Ways to ease the pain and stay mobile

Apart from following your doctor's orders or taking your therapist's advice there are a number of other things you can do to reduce your aches and pains and keep active. Doing something to help yourself is important because it goes hand in hand with the way you deal with your illness and the effect it may have on your life.

Although some forms of rheumatic disorders get better on their own, given time, others may not. That does not mean there will not be an effective way of controlling your illness, or that it will not come and go, giving you good days and not-so-good ones. You may have to accept that you are stuck with arthritis and that it will always be part of your life.

Coming to terms with this is easier said than done. The process may take you through the same range of emotions people experience when someone they love dies. That is because you are grieving; for the person you were before the illness struck, for the loss of all the things you used to be able to do.

At first you may feel a sense of shock, followed by anger and resentment. Why, you may ask, did this happen to me? Next come the black days, days when you feel depressed and frustrated.

All of these feelings are normal under the circumstances and it is important to acknowledge them, rather than try to deny them or hide the way you feel. Finding out about your illness, talking about it, crying - all of these things can help you move on to the next stage when you can begin to accept what has happened and move on from there.

Inevitably there will still be times when you feel angry, sad or depressed, but learning to accept things the way they are will help you make the most of life, despite your limitations. Instead of dwelling on the way

Mind over matter

Professor Dieppe, professor of rheumatology at the Bristol Royal Infirmary in the UK, says: "You may have pain, you may feel awful at times, you may think you look awful. But you mustn't let it become a disaster. No-one is interested in your becoming a martyr to arthritis.

"For a full and fulfilling future you need to relax into it, find ways round the problems, keep up with your family and friends and keep smiling. Talk about arthritis, share it with others, but never let it take over."

things were in the past, or thinking about the way things might have been, you can start to look forward to what you can do instead. Finding ways to help yourself deal with your illness and thinking positively about it is an important part of this process.

Pain relief

When you are in pain it can be extremely difficult to take a positive approach to life. So what else can you try, besides painkillers or other medication your doctor may have prescribed, to make things easier for yourself? There are a number of different approaches that have helped people. Some of these are listed below.

TENS

TENS, or transcutaneal electrical nerve stimulation, to give it its full title, stimulates the brain into producing its own painkillers: endorphins. It works by using low frequency electric signals and can be particularly helpful for people dealing with back or knee pain.

You simply strap on the battery-powered unit, which looks like a small box, making sure the contact points are over the painful area before you switch on. Pain relief is usually only temporary, but since the machine is portable you can go out and about wearing one.

TENS machines are quite expensive to buy but you may be able to borrow one from your doctor or physiotherapist to try out before you part with your cash. They don't work for everyone and should not be used by anyone who has a cardiac pacemaker. You shouldn't use the machine while you are driving a car or operating heavy machinery.

Acupuncture

In China, they have been practising acupuncture for more than 2,000 years, and an increasing number of Western doctors are now using it, particularly to help relieve

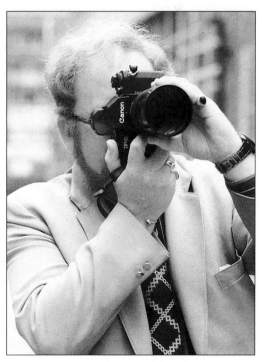

In spite of their arthritis, many people lead normal working lives, controlling their condition with pain killers and other medication. However, in the UK, arthritis costs around 88 million lost working days each year.

Taking control

pain. Fine, hair-like needles are inserted at key points on the body. This, it is thought, releases endorphins, which intercept the pain messages sent to the brain.

Most acupuncturists work privately, so you may have to pay if you want to try this kind of treatment. However, some doctors also practise acupuncture and your doctor may be able to refer you. For more information on finding a practitioner, turn to page 79 at the back of this book.

Hot and cold treatments

Simple hot and cold remedies can help relieve pain. Hot water bottles are one obvious example. Heat lamps work in much the same kind of way. Electric blankets can also be helpful, particularly the kind that can be left on overnight.

You can also buy pads at your local chemist or drugstore. Some, containing silica gel, can be heated by being placed in warm water and then applied to the joints. Others give off heat when they are opened up, because of a controlled chemical reaction. However this kind cannot be reused.

Ice packs placed over painful joints can also help ease pain; but if you keep the ice

Applying ice packs

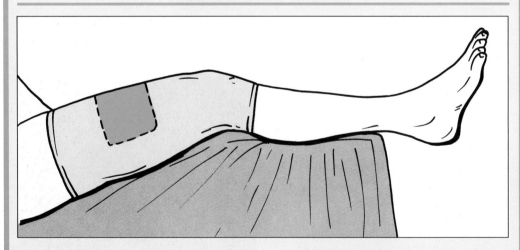

An ice pack is an effective and simple method of relieving pain. Never place them directly against the skin; always put a towel or some fabric in between. Elevate the affected limb and apply the ice pack for 10 minutes. Do not leave it on for longer. If you do not have an ice pack, you can use a packet of frozen peas instead.

packs in the freezer be careful not to place them directly against the skin as extreme cold can be as damaging as extreme heat. Always put a towel or other fabric in between the ice pack and your skin. It's worth remembering that a bag of frozen peas can always be used as an effective substitute for an ice pack.

Rest and exercise

Exercise is important, not only to stop joints stiffening up but also to keep muscles strong. If your joints get stiff and your muscles weak, you will end up putting too much strain on other parts of your body and exacerbating your problems.

Rest and exercise tips

● **Little and often is the key**
A little regular exercise every day is better than prolonged sessions less frequently. This applies to everyday activities, too. So do the heavy housework or gardening in short bursts, interrupted by short rests.

● **Time it right**
It is difficult to exercise when you are in pain. Time your sessions so that your pain killers are working and you are not too stiff or too tired.

● **Listen to your body**
If the exercises leave you in pain that lasts for a long time, you may be trying to do too much, too fast. It is important not to overdo things.

● **Reward yourself**
Try to make your sessions as pleasurable as possible. Play your favourite tapes or give yourself a treat afterwards. See if there are any exercises that you can do in a nice, warm bath.

● **Don't give up**
Even if you don't seem to be making much progress to begin with, keep at it. Make exercising an essential part of your daily life and routine, like cleaning your teeth, and it will soon become a habit.

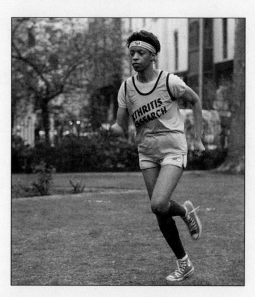

Taking control

It is difficult to generalise about the kind of exercise programme you should work out for yourself as the basic rules differ from one kind of rheumatic disorder to the next, and the balance between rest and exercise will vary depending on the type of illness you have and the stage it is at. For people with rheumatoid arthritis, for instance, rest is far more important than for people with osteoarthritis – particularly when in the middle of a flare-up.

You should always seek professional help before starting any exercise programme to make sure it is suitable for your particular condition. The best people to talk to are your doctor, physiotherapists and occupational therapists.

Protecting your joints

Inflamed or damaged joints need looking after, so you may have to re-think the way you do even simple things and everyday tasks.

A physiotherapist or occupational therapist may suggest that you wear splints to support or rest your joints. What else can you do?

Limber up at the start of the day

It can be helpful to start the day with some limbering up exercises so that you are loosened up before the morning begins. You can do these exercises either before you get out of bed or before you get dressed.

Start from your feet and work slowly up, repeating each movement about ten times. Don't rush – take it slowly. If you are very stiff in the mornings it might help to have a warm bath or shower first. You can exercise your hands in a basin of warm water.

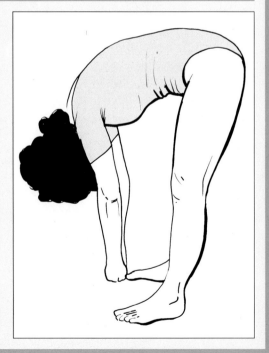

- Circle your ankles round and round and up and down as fully as possible.
- Bend your knees as far as you can and straighten them out.
- Do the same for your fingers, wrists and elbows.
- Stretch your arms above your head.
- Roll your head gently from side to side.

● Protect your hands by avoiding heavy lifting or gripping. Always use two hands instead of one whenever it is possible.

● Protect your hips and knees by adjusting the height of your bed and chairs so they are easy to get out of. Try not to go up and down stairs unnecessarily.

● Choose clothes that are easy to put on and take off, and wear lightweight shoes that support your feet without squashing them.

● Re-organise your daily routines. What tasks can you avoid altogether? Could you let the dishes drip dry instead of using a tea towel? What tasks can you make easier for yourself? Could you afford a dishwasher? What tasks can you delegate? Why not ask your children to do the washing up?

● Pace yourself. Instead of doing all the ironing at once, for example, set yourself a time limit, then stop and rest. Do a little more later or another day.

Relaxation method

Many people find themselves caught in a vicious circle of pain and stress. It works like this: the more pain you feel, the more stressed you become, the more you worry about pain, the more pain you feel and so on. Stress can make your muscles even tighter and more tense and as a result can make you less likely to feel able to get on top of your illness.

One way of breaking the circle is to teach yourself the skill of relaxation. Setting aside just twenty minutes a day to fight against tension can bring enormous benefits.

The more you practise relaxing, the better you will get. There are a number of tapes and booklets which can help you, or you could try the method outlined below.

● Chose a time when you won't be interrupted and find a quiet place.

● Lie down so that you are as comfortable as possible.
● Close your eyes and concentrate on your body, becoming aware of your breathing.
● Empty your mind as much as possible, Try to ignore any sounds around you.
● Begin to feel the tension flowing out of you.
● Concentrate on your toes and feet. Tighten up the muscles there and then relax them as much as you can.
● Feel the difference between the tension and the floppiness.
● Move up your body slowly, to your lower legs and knees. Repeat the 'tighten and relax' process.
● Slowly move on, working your way right up to your scalp, taking each part of your body in turn.
● Now take deep slow breaths. Let your mind and body sink into total relaxation.

Taking control

Angry cat

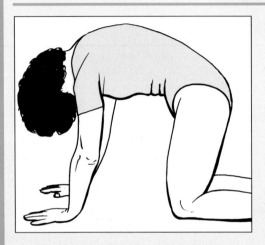

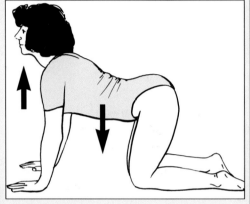

1 Kneel down on all-fours with your palms flat on the floor and your arms straight. Breathe in and arch your back upwards.

2 Hold the position for a few seconds, then breathe out and slowly lower your back to the original starting position. Repeat. This exercise will help increase mobility in your back.

Back arch

Lie down on the floor on your stomach and slowly raise your upper body off the floor, bending your elbows with your lower arms flat on the floor.

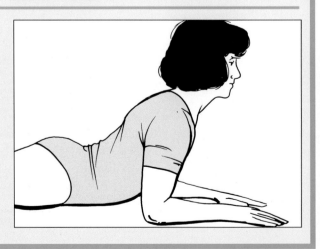

Lower back stretch

Lie on your back with your knees bent and feet flat on the floor. Raise one leg off the floor and, clasping your knee, bring it in towards your chest while you lift your head and shoulders off the floor. Lower slowly and then repeat with the other leg.

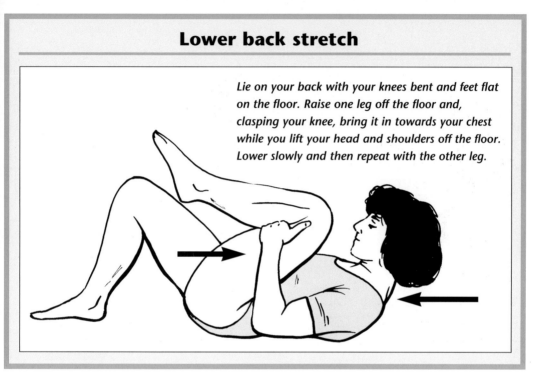

Pelvic tilting

Lie on your back on the floor with your knees bent and your feet flat on the floor. Clasp your hands across your stomach and then press the small of your back into the floor, pulling your stomach muscles in as you do so.

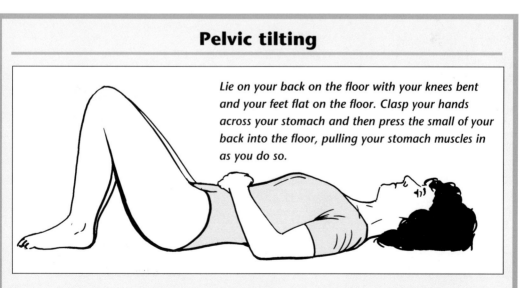

Taking control

Back and leg roll

1 *Lie on your back with your feet flat on the floor, knees bent and arms at your sides.*
2 *Now lift your feet off the floor and clasp your hands behind your knees.*
3 *Pull your knees in towards your chest. Hold for a few seconds and then roll your knees* *over to one side, rolling from the hips only and keeping your back flat on the floor. Roll over to the other side and then return to the original position. Like all these exercises, if you experience any pain or numbness, stop immediately.*

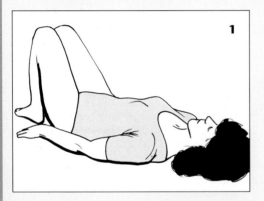

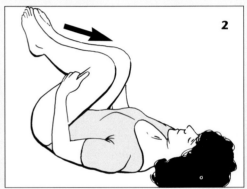

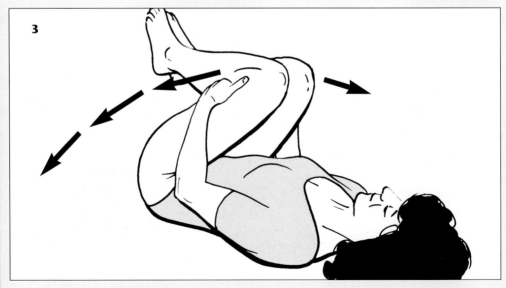

Achilles stretch

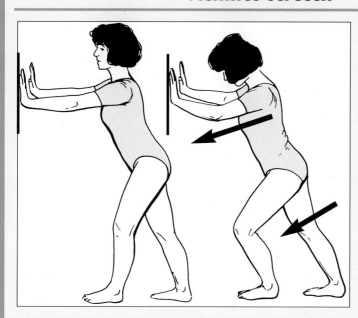

Stand at arms' length away from a wall and place your palms flat on the wall with arms straight and outstretched. Place one leg in front of the other. Now bend the knee of the leg in front and stretch out the leg behind you, keeping your heels flat on the floor, and bending your elbows slightly and pushing against the wall with your hands. Hold the stretch and then repeat with the other leg.

Back and thigh stretch

Lie on your back and bend your knees with your legs curled up beside you. Stretch your arms back behind your head. Feel the stretch in your thighs, back and shoulders. Hold for a few seconds and then release.

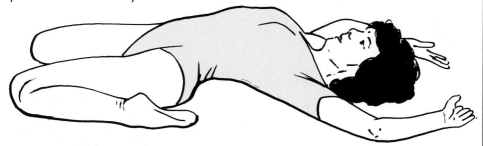

Taking control

Leg swings

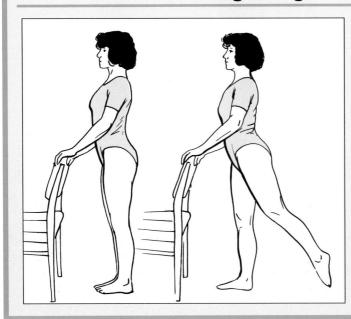

1 Stand up straight facing the back of a chair and holding on to it with your hands.
2 Keeping the supporting leg straight, raise your other leg off the floor and swing it back behind you. Hold and then return to the original position. Swing the leg back 3 times and then repeat with the other leg.

Knee flexing

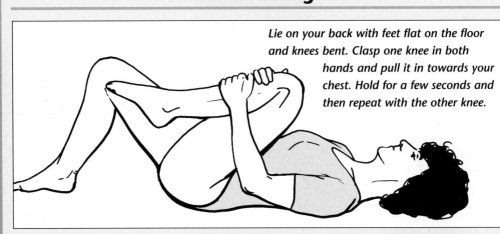

Lie on your back with feet flat on the floor and knees bent. Clasp one knee in both hands and pull it in towards your chest. Hold for a few seconds and then repeat with the other knee.

Back, leg and hip mobilizer

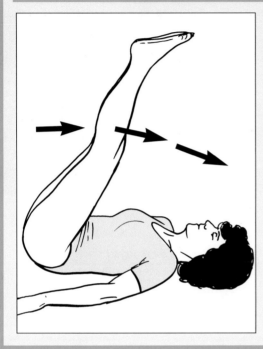

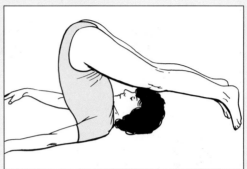

1 Lie on your back with arms out to the sides.
2 Slowly and gently lift your legs and then your hips and back off the floor and slowly extend your legs back over your head until your feet touch the floor behind you. Hold this body stretch as long as feels comfortable, and then slowly unwind and roll back down towards the floor, and relax.

Leg lifts

Lie on your stomach with your head resting on your arms. Lift one leg slowly off the floor and raise it as high as feels comfortable. Lower it to the floor and then repeat with the other leg.

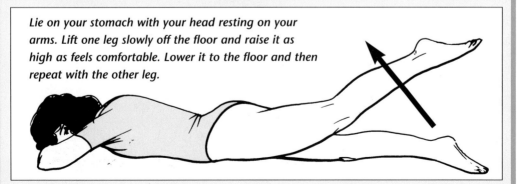

Taking control

Hip mobilizers

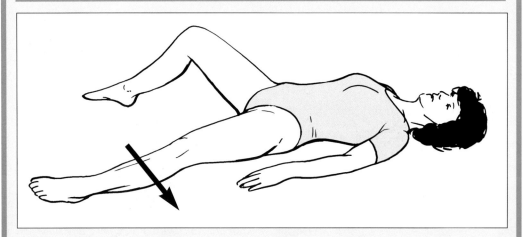

Lie on your back on the floor with your arms at your sides and your legs apart. Gently move your legs further apart, as far as feels comfortable. Hold the stretch for a few seconds and then slowly return your legs to the starting position in the centre.

Shoulder circling

Stand or sit up straight with elbows bent and your hands resting lightly on your shoulders or on the back of your neck. Now circle your upper arms backwards from the shoulders. Repeat 5 times and then change direction and rotate them forwards 5 times.

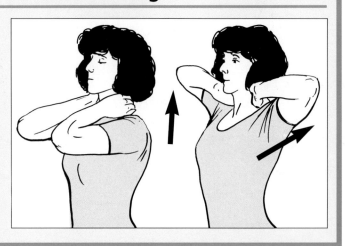

Arm raises

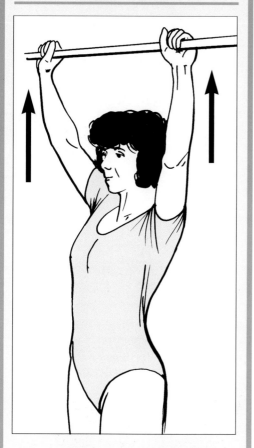

Hold a broomstick or long pole in both hands across your chest, and then extend your arms upwards, raising the stick up above your head. Hold for a few seconds and then lower it down to your chest. Repeat several times.

Arm swings

Stand up straight, legs shoulder distance apart, and slowly swing your arms back behind you. Hold the stretch and then return to the starting position. Swing them back several times.

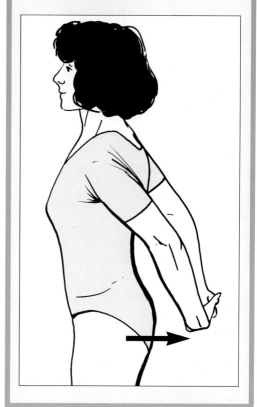

Taking control

Neck stretches

Raise one arm over your head as you lower your head down to rest on your shoulder. Feel the stretch in your neck on the other side. Hold the stretch for as long as feels comfortable, then return to the centre. Repeat to the other side.

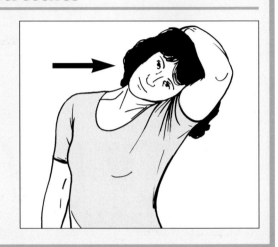

Arm chops

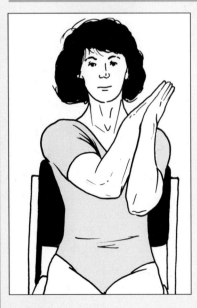
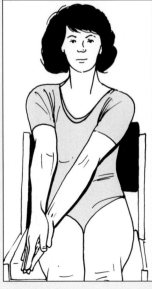

1 Sit up straight on a chair with your elbows bent and palms pressed together pointing over your left shoulder.
2 Chop your hands sharply downwards towards your right knee, straightening your arms as you do so. Repeat the exercise on the other side.

Palm presses

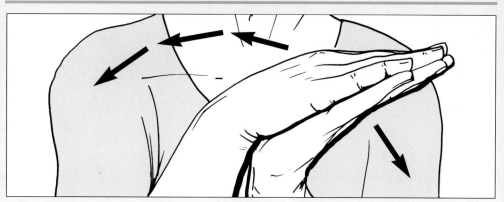

1 Place one hand on top of the other with the palms pressed together.
2 Reverse the lower hand over the top one and press down hard on the other side. This helps increase wrist flexibility and restores the range of movements.

Wrist stretches

Do this stretch over the edge of a table. Place one hand on the edge with the wrist bent and fingers pointing downwards. Use your other hand to help lift your hand up, stretching as far as it will go so that your fingers point upwards. Do this exercise several times and then repeat with the other hand.

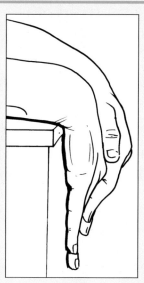
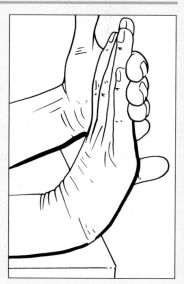

Taking control

Finger mobility exercises

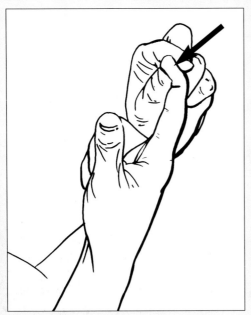

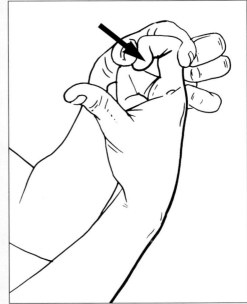

These exercises will help increase the flexibility and mobility of your fingers and hands. Stretch out your fingers and fingertips, one joint at a time, using your other hand to help bend and straighten the joints and stretch out the fingers. Work on the knuckle joints as well as the finger joints, curling and uncurling your hands. Bend your fingers back, one at a time, against your other hand, and gently pull your fingers outwards.

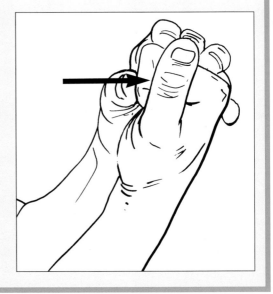

Joint hypermobility

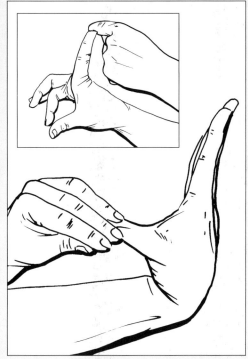

Only about five per cent of people have joint hypermobility. They are particularly supple and some, or all, of their joints are capable of a wide range of movement. Sometimes these people may be susceptible to problems with their joints. For instance, they may feel pain in their joints and the surrounding muscles after exercising.

If this happens to you, try taking paracetamol(an analgesic) or ibuprofen(an NSAID). Both can be purchased over the counter without a doctor's prescription. Instead of just taking them to relieve the pain after exercise, try taking them 30 minutes before you start exercising. If these do not help, ask your doctor to prescribe a stronger tablet with a longer-lasting action.

Physiotherapy and gentle stretching(as in the exercises featured in this chapter) may also help. Physiotherapists may recommend slow, static contractions through the full range of movement, or stretching the muscles and ligaments around the painful joints.

Just because you have hypermobile joints and may feel pain around these joints, it does not mean that you have arthritis or a disease of the joints. Only a small proportion of people go on to develop osteoarthritis. You may get fluid in the joints or even a dislocated joint, such as a hip, shoulder or knee. The symptoms may be very similar to those of arthritis and there is a danger that you may not be taken seriously when you complain of pain or stiffness.

However, for some people there are advantages in being hypermobile, particularly if they are athletes or dancers. Body flexibility can help improve sporting performance although it may also predispose athletes to dislocation of joints and stretching of ligaments. It is a good idea to avoid over-use of hypermobile joints for this reason. If you enjoy sport, swimming and cycling are both excellent forms of physical exercise.

Taking control

Lifting and bending

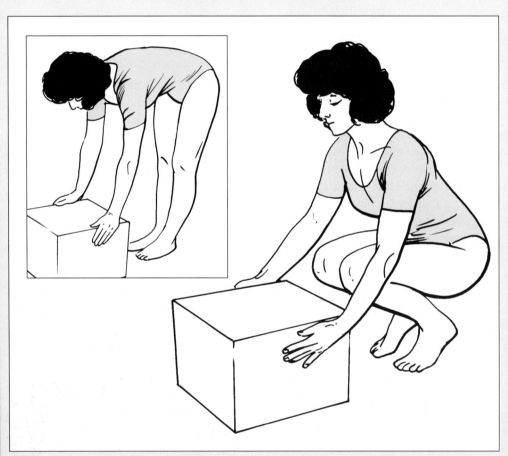

Never lift a heavy object by leaning over from the waist with your legs straight (as shown inset). Always bend your knees when lifting something off the ground or from a level beneath you. Keeping the object close to your body, rise with it, taking the strain on your leg muscles, not your back.

Chapter five
Home and away

Adapting your lifestyle

Your illness may mean that you can no longer do all the things you would like, but the trick is not to give up too soon. With a little ingenuity it is often possible to find a different way of doing things altogether.

People with rheumatic disorders have to adapt their lifestyle in order to suit their circumstances but there are many changes that can be made that will help both in the home and out and about.

An occupational therapist can be an invaluable source of help and advice and there are many useful booklets published by specialist organisations. For more information on these, turn to the list of useful addresses at the back of this book (see page 79).

In the home

You may want to put in a downstairs toilet or refit your kitchen and bathroom to make life easier. However, not all changes need be so drastic or expensive. Even little things can make a big difference – training members of your family to put things back where they belong, for instance, can cut down on the amount of lifting and carrying you have to do.

Rethinking the way you store things can help, too. Make sure that the things you use often, or things that are fragile or heavy, are in easy reach rather than tucked away in awkward spaces or stored in cupboards that are overhead or below waist height and may involve stretching, reaching and bending.

Long-reach aids or 'grabbers' can be invaluable and it may be worth having several. Keep one hanging in each place where you are most likely to need help; this saves

you having to go back and forth to get one.

You could think about having your power points moved up the walls so that you don't have to bend down to the skirting

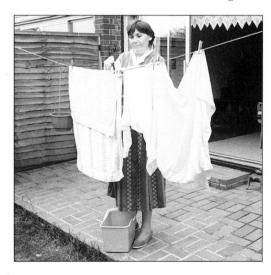

board every time you want to plug in an iron or a vacuum cleaner. Phone points need not be at floor level either. An alternative to moving the power points would be to use an extension socket – however be careful about trailing flexes.

Special plugs with built-in handles are easier to pull out than conventional ones. Rocker switches are easier to switch off and on than ones that have to be flicked up and down. Time switches may also be useful.

It is also easier to open a door with a lever handle than one that has a round knob and has to be gripped and turned. Remember also that sliding windows are easier to open than sash ones.

Other thoughts? You could fit a pulley cord to your curtains and a wire basket behind your letter box. You might want to put up extra hand rails on the stairs to help you. For housework, use a long-handled dust pan and brush, and a long mop.

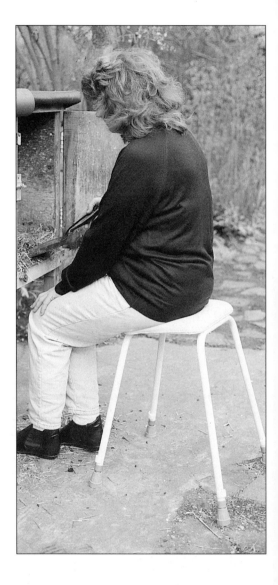

Many people find that it is easier to perform quite simple tasks about the house and garden if they are sitting down at the right level rather than having to bend over. You can purchase a special lightweight stool which is easy to carry around.

In the kitchen

It is probably a good idea to rearrange your cupboards so that all the things you use regularly are within easy reach. Ideally everything would be on one level, but this tends to be impossible in practice. Even so, you can minimize lifting, bending and

Making life easier around the house

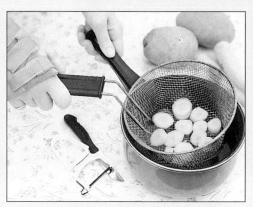

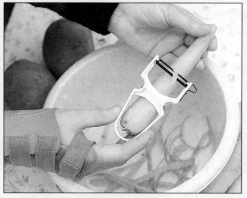

To avoid lifting heavy saucepans, especially when containing hot liquids, you can use a wire basket with a handle to lower vegetables and other foods for boiling or frying into the saucepan.

You can use a specially designed peeler for peeling carrots, potatoes and other vegetables and fruit. This can be pulled along the vegetable to remove the peel without having to curl your fingers round it.

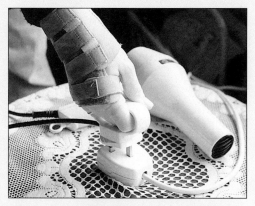

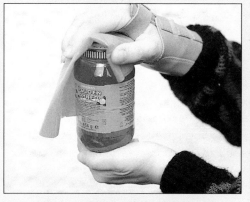

Plugs with a built-in handle are easier to fit into adaptors and sockets, and to pull out, than conventional ones. Fit them to the electrical appliances you use most.

A special plastic sheet which grips the lids of jars and bottles makes opening them much easier when your hands are swollen and painful.

Home and away

carrying heavy objects. A heat-proof trivet next to the stove would probably be useful to avoid carrying heavy pans and casseroles.

You could keep together in one place those items you always use at the same time: for example, milk, sugar, tea, coffee, kettle and mugs. Instead of carrying the kettle to the sink, think about topping it up with water from a light-weight jug.

Other handy gadgets to think about include bottle top turners and kettle tippers long-handled squeegee mops and dustpans can help make cleaning less of a chore.

You might consider whether it is worth replacing your saucepans with lightweight ones, preferably non-stick to make washing up easier. A flip-top rubbish bin may be better for you than one operated by a foot pedal, and one that swings out and opens up from beneath a work surface when you open a cupboard door may be better still.

Think about fitting baskets and shelves

> ## Making life easier
>
> Make everything as easy as possible for yourself. If your hands are painful, use sliced bread and spreads that are soft even when they come straight from the fridge. Do you really have to peel potatoes, or could you bake them in their jackets or boil them in their skins and peel them later?

on the back of doors for storage. Hooks can be used to hang tools and gadgets within easy reach.

Think, too, about the way you do the chores. Instead of taking a saucepan to the sink to drain the vegetables, you could cook them in a lift-out wire mesh basket like the ones used for frying potato chips. Then you only have the weight of the water to carry.

In the bathroom

Showers may be easier to manage than having a bath, but soaking in a hot tub can ease aches and pain. Bath rails can help you get in and out and a non-slip bath mat is a *must*. Some people find a bath board or seat a good idea.

If you think that having a shower would be less of a struggle than having a bath, do seek the advice of your doctor or an occupational therapist before you go ahead and get a shower installed specially.

Walk-in showers may be easier to

manage than the kind that have a raised edge to the tray at the bottom. A bidet might also be worth considering.

If you find it difficult to get up and down from the toilet you can get a seat raise. A grab rail might help, too, Toilets can also be adapted so that they are easier to flush. If your bathroom is on the first floor and you find going up and downstairs a problem, you might consider a discreet commode.

Washing and drying yourself can be difficult if you find it hard to stretch or bend. Some people find it's better washing with a sponge than a flannel because the soap lathers up more easily. Long-handled back brushes can be used to reach other extremities - you can wrap the flannel round the bristles for a gentler touch.

Fixing the nail brush to the wall means you take your hands to the brush, not the other way round.

Wrapping yourself in a large bath sheet may be the easiest way to dry off – or you could slip into a towelling robe. Wriggling your toes on a bath mat or towel is a way of drying your feet if you can't reach them.

In the bedroom

Duvets or continental quilts may be easier to manage than blankets which have to be tucked in, although you may have to get someone else to change the covers. If you really prefer blankets, lightweight cellular ones are probably best.

A firm bed is best for the joints but this does not have to be an expensive 'orthopaedic' one. Pine beds often have wooden slats under the mattress which provide a firm base. You may even be able to put a board between the base and the mattress of your present bed. Raising the height of your bed may make it easier to get in and out. You can purchase special bed blocks for this purpose.

Make sure that you can reach your clothes easily. Lightweight sliding baskets may be better than heavy drawers for storage. You may want to fit hanging rails in your wardrobe which can be pulled out (rather like towel rails in kitchens) for easier access.

When buying clothes, go for lightweight items. Several lighter layers tend to be warmer than one thick one anyway. You can get special aids to help you dress: devices to pull up zip fasteners, do up buttons and ease on tights (panty hose).

Before you buy

Before you buy extra equipment, consider the pros and cons carefully. Would a food processor really be worth the expense? They are heavy and need more washing up than a simple sharp knife. On the other hand an electric can opener fixed to the wall might be a boon, and a microwave oven might be easier than working with a conventional one.

Would it be easier if you had a shallower sink – or a smaller washing up bowl? Lever taps are the easiest to operate and a swivel spout may let you stand a saucepan next to the sink and fill it without having to hold it as it fills up with water.

Home and away

In the living room

You will need a suitable chair – one that is high enough for you to get up and down from without too much strain, and which provides good back support. When you are sitting you should be able to rest your feet on the floor. You can get chairleg extenders to raise the height and a board under the seat cushion can make the base firmer. You can also buy special riser chairs but it is a good idea to test these out before you buy to make sure the model you fancy is the right one for you; otherwise you could find yourself living with a very expensive mistake.

Most telephones have push button controls these days, which are certainly easier to use than the old dials. The models do vary, though, and you may find the ones with bigger buttons easier to use. Contact your phone company for details of the services and products they provide for the disabled.

Fitting an intercom for your front door may save you unnecessary journeys. Having a television set with a remote control device could make it easier to change channels from your chair without having to struggle to your feet.

If you do not have a telephone with push-button controls, you could try inserting a pen or pencil in the dial to make dialling easier. However, it may be worth looking at other models with larger push-buttons. Contact the sales department of your phone company for advice.

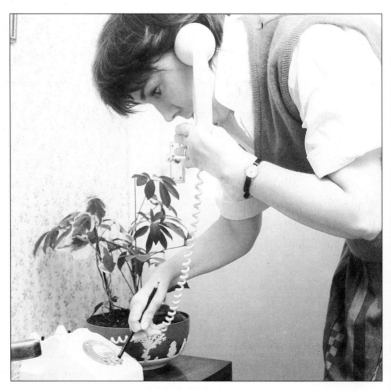

Out and about

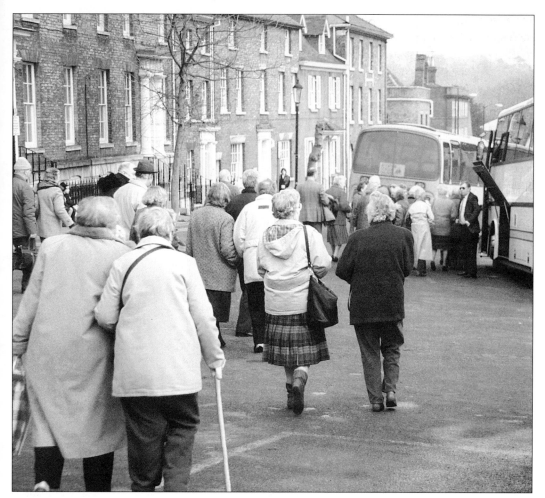

At least in your own home you can reorganise things to make your life easier. However, once you step beyond your front door things are less likely to be under your control.

If you are not entirely fit and mobile then there is no doubt that public transport is anything but user friendly. So if you have to travel by bus, train, tube or plane, it is always worth planning your journey well in advance so you can work out how best to cope.

You can obtain some more detailed information and helpful advice on how to get about from the organisations listed at the back of this book (see page 79).

Home and away

Walking aids

Not all walking sticks are the same and although in the UK some are available on the National Health Service you might find it pays to buy one that will suit you better. You need to be sure that the length is right for you and that you can hold the handle comfortably. Make sure that you are shown how to use your stick properly (there are some basic guidelines) so that it gives you the support you need.

A walking stick should always have a rubber end on the bottom: to grip the pavement and prevent the stick slipping. Replace this rubber end as soon as it gets worn.

Even if you do not like the idea of using a stick because it makes you feel awkward or self-conscious, it does have some advantages over and above the extra support it gives. Other people are more likely to give you a little consideration. It is a clue to motorists that you won't be able to break into a run if the lights change when you are halfway across a pedestrian crossing.

Wheelpower

If you cannot always get around on your own two feet, even with the aid of a stick or a frame, then you will need to investigate the possibilities of wheelpower. Once again, you should get expert advice. Although in Britain it is easier to obtain a self-propelled wheelchair on the National Health Service than a powered one, these can be difficult to use if you have weak hands or shoulders - and learning to push a wheelchair is not as easy as it might seem, either!

A powered wheelchair or scooter (and there are many on the market) is likely to be expensive but will probably make you feel more independent. Another possibility might be an electrically powered bicycle or trike. There are some companies that specialize in adapting bikes and trikes for disabled people.

However, for many people the ideal solution is a car of their own, adapted if necessary for their needs. Not all conversions are expensive, but if a car needs an almost total refit, this is bound to be costly.

For more information on wheelchairs, electrically powered bicycles and cars, and a list of useful organisations and addresses, turn to the section at the back of this book (see page 79).

Children with arthritis

Many parents cannot believe it when they learn that their child has arthritis; they often think that it is an old people's disease. However, children can be affected too, and one in 1,000 children suffers from juvenile arthritis during their early years.

So why do these children get arthritis? Research is being carried out, but we still don't understand the exact reasons. There is no medical evidence that it is genetic, inherited, connected with a virus infection, as a result of poor diet or catching cold or sleeping in a damp bed – all theories that have been expounded, but without any firm proof. There are several types of juvenile arthritis, which may start in different ways.

Systemic arthritis

This form of arthritis affects boys and girls, especially those who are under five. The child develops a fever and a rash. It usually begins like an infection with a persistent high temperature, which may last days or even weeks. The child has a fever at night although it often subsides by lunchtime the following day, only to return at night. The child becomes listless and progressively weaker, may lose weight and become anaemic.

He may also have a red, blotchy rash and enlarged glands in the neck, under the arms and in the groin. The limbs will ache and there will be discomfort in the joints, although no swelling.

Many children do make a full recovery from systemic arthritis after several months or even more than a year, but a few have problems with persistent or recurrent arthritis.

Polyarthritis

Girls are more likely than boys to develop this type of arthritis, which can occur at any age and even affect babies of a few months. It usually starts very suddenly and without warning: a number of joints become painful and inflamed, sometimes in rapid succession. The child becomes tired, apathetic and unwilling to use his limbs.

He will need to rest and may curl up with his joints in a bad position. For example, his knees could stiffen and this could adversely affect walking. Rest splints are sometimes used to hold wrists and knees in a good position.

Pauci-articular arthritis

This affects about two-thirds of children with arthritis. It might affect just one joint, usually the knee, and this is known as monarticular arthritis. This is more common in two or three-year-olds, often after a fall. The joint may start to swell after a minor injury. Sometimes, other joints get affected, e.g. the other knee, an ankle, an elbow or a finger. This is pauci-articular arthritis.

continued on page 68

Home and away

continued from page 67

Eye disease occurs in approximately one-third of children with this type of arthritis, and if your child is affected, it is important that he should have an eye test. His eyes should be checked by an ophthalmologist (eye specialist) using a slit lamp. Failure to diagnose this eye disease(chronic iridocyclitis) could lead to serious eye problems in the future and even blindness.

Juvenile spondylitis

This form of arthritis is quite rare, and usually affects boys over nine years of age. It starts with inflammation of the joints in the legs, e.g. the knees, ankles and hips. Later the sacro-iliac joints in the lower back may also become inflamed. Another type of eye disease is associated with this form of arthritis: acute iridocyclitis. A child may get a painful, red eye; if this happens, an eye specialist should be consulted.

This form of arthritis may be inherited. Children usually carry a special genetic factor(HLA-B27), and other family members may suffer from ankylosing spondylitis, spinal stiffness or eye problems. However, although you may have this tissue type(genetic factor) you will not necessarily develop arthritis; only a minority do.

Adult-type rheumatoid arthritis

This arthritis of the small joints in the hands and feet, and coccasionally the knees and elbows, affects mainly girls over eleven years of age. It can be detected by a blood test, and long-acting drugs are used to treat and manage the disease to prevent serious damage to the joints.

Psoriatic arthritis

With this type of arthritis, there is scaling of the skin. Although usually mild, it is often recurrent. However, in a minority of cases it can be severe and widespread, and will need special drug therapy to treat it.

Leading a normal life

Most children with arthritis still go to school and lead a relatively normal life. They usually have stiff, painful joints in the mornings and may need to exercise and have a warm bath before leaving for school. Their symptoms can vary from day to day, and some days will be worse than others. Teachers should be made aware of the child's arthritis so that they can look out for the signs of pain and tiredness. Often children may be quiet and withdrawn, behave badly or be unwilling to join in games – these are all indications that the child may be in pain.

● A child may need to stand up and walk around between lessons to relieve stiffness after sitting at a desk for a long time.

● He may need to avoid body-contact sports, and perhaps do his own special exercise programme instead, which has been designed to keep the muscles strong and the joints mobile.

● He may need time off school for doctor's

and hospital appointments, for physiotherapy and hydrotherapy sessions.
● He should be encouraged to swim. Swimming is the most appropriate form of exercise as it helps develop strength and mobility without putting any weight on the joints.
● He may have to take medication at school to reduce pain and inflammation. If so, the teacher should be aware of this.
● He may even need time off for hospital tests or an operation.

If your child is affected, it is important that he should lead as normal a life as possible and should be treated normally by his family, teachers and peers. Most children want to lead independent lives and do things for themselves, even if it takes more time than usual to do simple things like walk up and down stairs, go to the lavatory, do up buttons, tie shoe laces and open doors.

You should discuss any special problems your child may have with his teacher. Let the school know if he requires special pencils, computers etc. It is also important that periods of illness or hospitalization interfere as little as possible with your child's schoolwork and academic development. If he needs time off school, it may be possible to arrange for a home tutor or a teacher in hospital.

Your child's diet

Some children with arthritis may be sensitive to certain foods such as milk, milk products and eggs. Although there is no evidence that special diets can be helpful in
continued on page 70

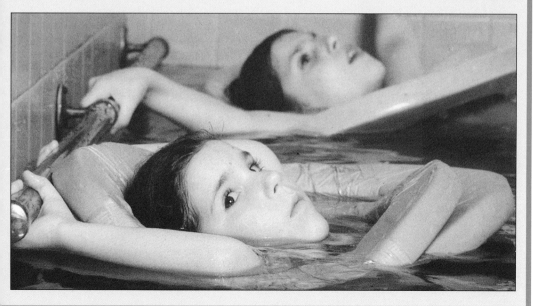

Home and away

contuinued from page 69
treating chronic arthritis, it is important that your child eats a healthy, balanced diet with an adequate calorie intake. Protein is very important for building strong muscles, as is calcium for strong bones.

Exercise

An exercise programme will probably be devised for your child by the physiotherapist, and you will be shown how to supervise these exercises at home. They are usually performed at least twice a day and will be designed to:

● Maintain the position and function of all joints, whether affected or unaffected by arthritis.

● To strengthen the muscles above and

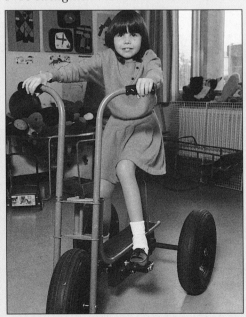

below the affected joints.

● To help the development of muscles.

● To increase mobility.

Exercising in a warm-water pool relaxes the muscles and enables movement of joints without putting any weight on them. At home, many of these exercises can be performed in a warm bath.

Walking may have to be kept to a minimum for young children with problems in their lower limb joints, and they may benefit from tricycles, pedal cars and other exercise toys which encourage muscles to develop normally without putting strain on inflamed joints.

Treatments

Unfortunately, there are no wonder drugs to cure arthritis, and usually anti-inflammatory drugs are used to manage the illness. Cortisone and steroid drugs may be used for treating very serious systemic illness, but are usually given only every other day, or no more than once a day. Because of their side effects, they must be used with great care; they can cause thinning of the bones, stunted growth and lower the resistance to infection.

Talk to your doctor about your child's medication and any possible side effects. It is important that you understand the treatment and what is involved. Don't be afraid to ask questions and get him to explain how and when the tablets or medicines should be taken.

Chapter six

Getting the most out of life

Leisure time and lifestyle

When you suffer from rheumatism or from arthritis, it can be all too easy to dwell on the things you cannot do, rather than making the most of the things you can. That is why keeping up your interests and hobbies, or developing new ones, is vital.

Illness puts an extra strain on your relationships and the difficulties can be compounded if you are feeling worthless or useless. Doing things you enjoy will improve your morale, boost your sense of self worth and help you look forward, not back.

Gardening

If you have never been much of a gardener, now could be the time to start. After all, you don't have to look after acres of ground to get pleasure out of seeing things grow; you can put tubs on the patio or pots on the windowsill.

On the other hand, if gardening has always been one of the pleasurable ways in which you have used your spare time, you might be worrying whether you will still be able to carry on. The good news is that you don't have to give up gardening, even if you can't manage all the heavy work.

Of course, you will have to rethink the way you organise your garden, rather like the way you may have to reorganise your home. There are specialist organisations to help you

and offer practical advice. For more detailed information turn to page 79.

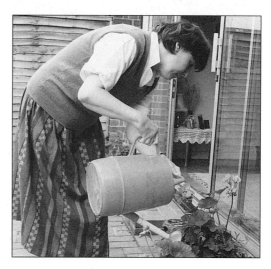

Getting the most out of life

Tips for gardeners

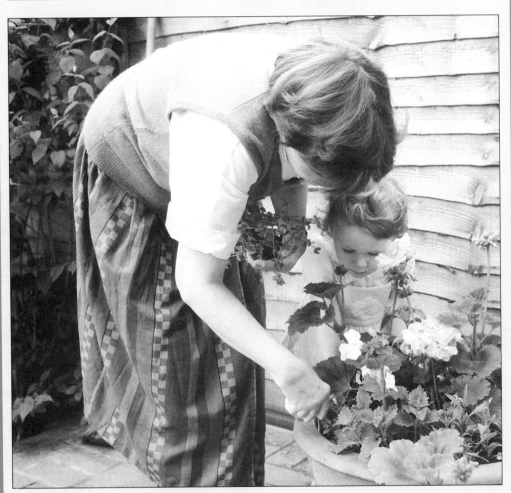

● Use plants that provide good ground cover, or lay bark chippings in borders to cut down on weeds.

● If mowing is a problem, think about replacing the lawn with a paved or gravel area.

● Raised flower beds not only look attractive, but you can work in them while you are sitting down.

● Long-handled lightweight garden tools are easier to use than conventional ones.

Reading

People often say that they never have time to sit down and read, but if your illness forces you to rest then you have the ideal excuse for rediscovering the world of books. Here are some tips to help make reading easier.

● Make the most of your local library or send for books by post

● Ask your occupational therapist about book rests and page turners if your hands are painful.

● Don't forget that there is now a wide range of books on tape, which you can listen to. Many libraries have a good range from which to choose.

Arts and crafts

You don't have to give these up. If you keep your fingers mobile you can sew, knit, paint or take up a host of other crafts. In fact, there are many specialist gadgets on the market which are widely available to help you. These include self-threading needles, tapestry kits, which have larger than usual holes, and battery-operated scissors.

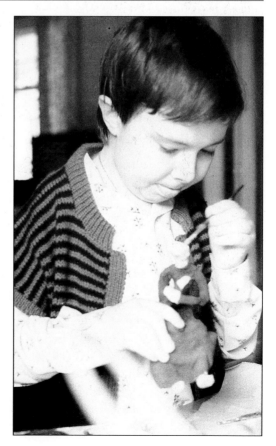

Getting the most out of life

Sport

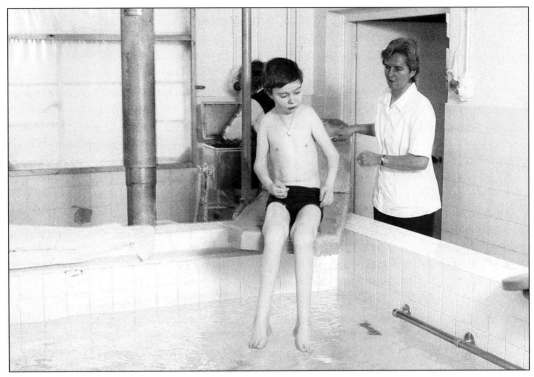

Even if you can no longer play energetic sports, such as tennis or golf you might still be able to take part in a different way, by becoming an umpire or a scorer or perhaps just a loyal spectator.

Swimming is the one sport you should try. In warm water you will be able to move stiff joints more freely and feel some easing of the pain. Find out if there are special sessions at your local pool, perhaps for adults only, or for disabled people. If you cannot swim there may be special adult learner classes. Why not enrol? Swimming is an excellent form of exercise, and it is very relaxing and enjoyable.

Swimming

This is an excellent form of exercise and therapy for adults and children alike. Swimming causes little pain and is actually very soothing as it relaxes muscles and aching joints. In the warm water of a heated swimming pool, joints can move more freely. Your doctor or consultant may recommend special exercises in a hydrotherapy pool.

Clubs and penpals

Broadening your social circle can be difficult if your illness restricts your mobility, but it is worth thinking about joining a self-help group or charity if only because that is one way to make new friends

If you want to get away from your illness altogether, think about joining a club or society connected with your favourite pastime or interests: the local poetry reading circle, for instance, or an environmental group or organisation. Your local library will be a good source of information about what goes on in your area, and you could always phone if you cannot get there. Some clubs are specifically for women and have local groups which meet in members homes to discuss anything from law and order to aromatherapy – anything, in fact, so long as it's not housework and childcare!

If you can't get out, let your fingers do the talking: become a penpal. If writing is hard, would a computer keyboard be easier to use? Or what about a club where you correspond by cassette? Some arthritis charities run pen clubs for this purpose. There are also specialist clubs for children and young people who suffer from arthritis. This helps them to make new friends on paper. Who knows? If they correspond a lot, they might meet up at some future date.

Relationships

Making new friends outside the family is one thing. Getting on with those at home is another. Living with people can be difficult at the best of times, however much you love them, and if you are not in the best of health than there is bound to be an extra strain on the relationship.

Because pain is not visible, like a rash or a broken leg, the people around you may not realise how you are feeling. They may not understand that things can change for you even from day to day, or from one week to the next.

Some people have days when they can get quite a lot done without too much trouble. At other times just getting up and getting dressed can take it out of them for the rest of the day.

It can be hard for others to understand the nature of your illness or how it may affect you. They may get impatient at times. They may even begin to treat you like a helpless child, which can be very upsetting and frustrating.

There will be some days when you need more help than others, and days when you want to do most things for yourself. It is quite likely you will find it hard to ask for help when you need it - or accept it when it is offered, especially if you have always been independent.

It is important for you to acknowledge

Getting the most out of life

the jumble of feelings you may have about all this. You need to talk about the way you feel with your partner and other family members. After all, they are not mind readers and unless you let them know how you feel and how best they can help you, then the relationships between you are likely to become more, not less, strained.

You and those closest to you are quite likely to find yourselves grappling with a whole range of negative emotions. You may worry about your illness making you a burden. You may secretly fear that the strain on your partner or the people who are closest to you might become so great that one day they will abandon you. You may

feel guilty or resentful about being needy.

They may feel guilty too – guilty about getting impatient or being thoughtless, guilty for thinking about themselves. They may feel resentful about the situation and there may even be times when they feel trapped.

All of these feelings are perfectly normal human reactions, but to counter them you will have to draw deeply on all the resources any relationship relies on, e.g. tolerance, compromise and, above all, communication.

If you find it too difficult to work through your problems together, don't be afraid to seek outside help. Some counsellors, for instance, are skilled at helping people through rocky patches and it may be possible

Making relationships better

● Try to separate the management of your day-to-day life from the management of your relationship. Both need attention, but don't muddle them up. Sort out the practical problems together and set aside a completely different time to talk about your feelings.
● Don't bottle things up. It is better to acknowledge and deal with your feelings – but not necessarily in the heat of the moment. Wait for a calmer time, and try to say what you really mean.
● Instead of accusing your partner, see if you can identify the feeling you had and use 'I' statements, not 'You' ones. Instead of saying "*You* should have done this or that..." you could say "*I* felt ..... when you

did such and such."
● Learn to listen. Don't assume you know what your partner is thinking; and try to spot the feelings that may lie underneath the words.
● Make times to share things together, even if they are different from before. Sharing interests and activities strengthens the bonds between you.
● Allow each other time and space to be alone sometimes.
● Encourage your partner to learn about your illness with you. The more you both know, the more you will both be able to understand the emotional aspects of your illness as well as the medical ones.

to arrange to see a counsellor in your own home if you are not sufficiently mobile to visit their office. Ask your doctor or the ARC if you live in the UK.

Sex

If you have always had a close and loving sexual relationship with your partner there is no reason why you cannot continue to enjoy the intimacy of making love. Of course, you may have to re-think this aspect of your life, in the same way that you may have to reorganise other areas, but it is worth remembering that love-making is not just about sexual intercourse, it is about giving and receiving pleasure.

Making love-making better

● Time it right. Choose to make love at the time of day when you know you will be most mobile and your joints the least stiff. You probably know the best time to tackle other household activities. Give your love life the same kind of priority.
● Make love when you know that your pain killers will be at their most active. Incidentally, frequent sexual activity can reduce pain by stimulating the body's own pain killers: endorphins.
● Keep warm. A bath beforehand may help loosen you up. If your bedroom is chilly think about making love somewhere warmer, like the living room.
● Experiment with different positions to find ones that are comfortable for you. You may feel better on your side, or sitting, rather than on your back. Use pillows to support and cushion painful joints. A foam wedge,

more conventionally used by people who read in bed, may help if you find it hard to raise your legs.
● Think about using sex aids. If you can't use your hands as much as you'd like, a vibrator could be the answer. If the idea of buying one embarrasses you, a body massager works the same way.
● Make the first move sometimes. If your partner is afraid of causing you more pain, they may think twice before doing or saying anything that might make you feel under pressure to make love. If you sometimes make the advances you let them know that sex is still important, and that you still find them desirable.

Whatever else you do, don't stop touching. We all need to be held close and told we are loved. Sometimes, though, our own feelings about ourselves can get in the way. If a woman's hands are swollen and

---

A better sex life

Having to look again at the way you make love may even help you and your partner reach new discoveries about what pleases each of you. You may find, despite everything, that the sexual side of your relationship becomes warmer and more satisfying than it was before.

Getting the most out of life

misshapen she may no longer want to use them lovingly to stroke her partner's cheek. A man who took pride in his strong physique might fear that no one could desire his arthritic body.

If you feel unlovable you may behave in a way that brings about what you most fear. Consciously or unconsciously you may draw back from physical contact, leaving your partner hurt and rejected. That is why it is important to acknowledge your feelings about your body, share those feelings with your partner, and then try to accept yourself the way you are.

Make the most of yourself. Even if you find it difficult to wash your hair or dress attractively it is worth the effort – caring for yourself is important. It can reaffirm and boost your own sense of worth and self-esteem. Living with rheumatism or arthritis can undermine your self-confidence, but you can fight back. You need not let your illness run your life or ruin your relationships. And if you find that hard to believe, this is what rheumatologist Paul Dieppe says: "If an elderly person gets arthritis that affects just the right knee, causing some pain and a bit of stiffness, it might not pose much of a problem. But the same arthritis in a young man who is embarking on a career as a professional footballer could be a disaster. The handicap would be much greater for the young man than for the pensioner. Or would it?

"Perhaps the young man would realise that it was silly to continue with a sporting career and turn to accountancy without any great regret, Perhaps the pensioner would find the knee discomfort the last straw and let it get him down to such an extent that it became a disproportionately large problem: we all see people fall into that trap.

"So the handicap is up to you in some ways. It is more than the pain and the frustration and the joints not working properly. It is how you let it run your life and what you let the arthritis do to you.

"That's why I always tell people: don't let the arthritis get on top and handicap you."

Useful addresses

The Arthritis and Rheumatism Council
This charity raises money solely to further research and knowledge into rheumatic diseases. ARC is sponsoring a major effort to find the cause and cure of these diseases, and is funding more than 300 short-term projects in hospitals, universities and laboratories. It supports 30 research units, and circulates regular reports to all NHS GPs and some hospital doctors. It funds 27 appointments of professors and lecturers in rheumatology, and finances 45 research fellowships and PhD studentships. It supports bursaries and scholarships for physiotherapists and occupational therapists.

ARC
Chesterfield, Derbyshire
S41 7TQ
Tel: 01246 558033

Arthritis Care
18 Stephenson Way
London NW1 2HD
Tel: 0171 916 1500
Helpline: 0800 289170

National Ankylosing Spondylitis Society
5 Grosvenor Crescent
London SW1X 7ER
Tel: 0171 235 8585

Fibromyalgia Support Group
8 Rochester Grove
Stockport SK7 4JD
Tel: 0161 483 3155

Lupus UK
51 North Street
Romford, Essex RN1 1BA
Tel: 01708 731251

Psoriasis Association
7 Milton Street
Northampton NN2 7JG
Tel: 01604 711129

Chartered Society of Physiotherapy
14 Bedford Row
London WC1R 4ED
Tel: 0171 242 1941

College of Occupational Therapists
6-8 Marshalsea Road
Southwark, London SE1 1HL
Tel: 0171 357 6480

British Homeopathic Association
27a Devonshire Street
London W1N 1RJ
Tel: 0171 935 2163

General Council and Register of Osteopaths
56 London Street
Reading, Berks RG1 4SQ
Tel: 01734 576585

British Chiropractic Asociation
29 Whitley Street
Reading, Berks RG2 0EG
Tel: 01734 757557

Disabled Living Foundation
380 Harrow Road
London W9 2HU
Tel: 0171 289 6111

Gardens for the Disabled Trust
Hayes Farmhouse
Hayes Lane
Peasmarsh
East Sussex TN31 6XR
Tel: 01424 882345

Disabled Drivers Association
Ashwellthorpe Hall
Ashwellthorpe
Norwich, Norfolk NR6 1EX
Tel: 01508 41449

Australia

Arthritis Foundation
PO Box 370
Darlinghurst
2029 Australia

USA

Arthritis Foundation
17 Executive Park Drive NE
Suite 480
Atlanta
Georgia
USA 30329

Index